WOO PELLET SMOKER GRILL

COOKBOOK

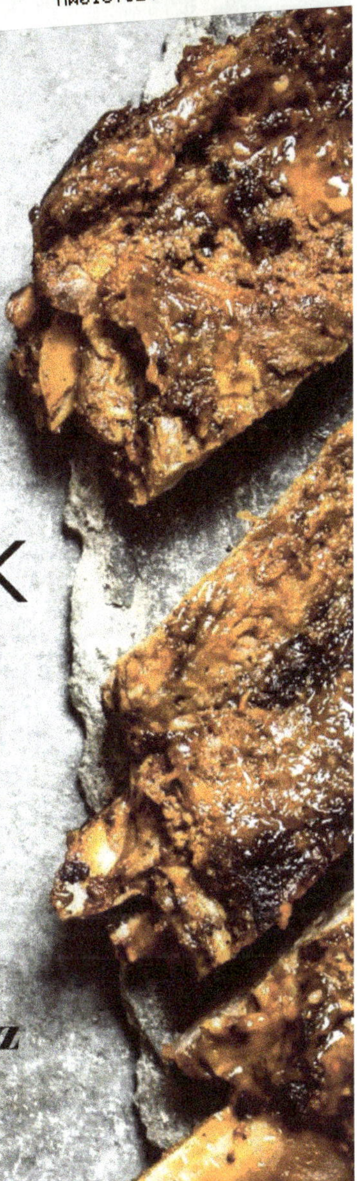

Miguel Gonzalez

2019-2020

Table of Contents

INTRODUCTION

Wood Pellet Smoker

It is a barbecue with grill that uses an electronic thermostat to feed the pellets; this allows to obtain a uniform heat and the cooking of the food is uniform.

The wood pellets used are not traditional, but a specific pellet is used for food in order not to pollute the food, also there are different types of pellets that are created from different types of wood.

Cooking with wood pellets smoker

Cooking with wood pellet smoker, means adding a touch more to the dish, in fact, the pellets chosen according to the wood used, enhance the taste of each dish making it unique and also are much healthier than charcoal and gas.

With them you can roast, cook, smoke and grill creating fantastic evenings with family or friends.

How it works

The product runs on electric current; by adding the pellets in the special hopper they arrive in a collector where a motor pushes them into the firebox according to the speed and time that has been set. Once the pellets have reached the firebox, the igniter creates a flame that starts to produce smoke around the grate until the set temperature is reached.

Advantages

One of the advantages to be taken into consideration, is the heating speed, in fact in maximum 10 minutes they are ready to be used; the second advantage is that they use an indirect cooking method that allows to roast, as in an oven. Thanks to this cooking, the products are never directly in contact with the heat source, and it is possible to make tasty low heat recipes.

The third advantage, is given by the flavours released by the dishes; thanks to these new barbecues and thanks to the pellets, the dishes take on a fantastic flavour of smoked wood having the possibility to choose to use different types of pellets created with different types of wood such as: maple, cherry, alder, walnut.

In this book you will find 100 tasty recipes to make with your wood pellet smoker;

Are you ready?

To start out check the best healthy 100 wood pellet smoker and grill recipes.

POURTY RECIPES FOR WOOD PELLET SMOKER GRILLS POULTRY

SMOKED BOURBON & ORANGE BRINED TURKEY

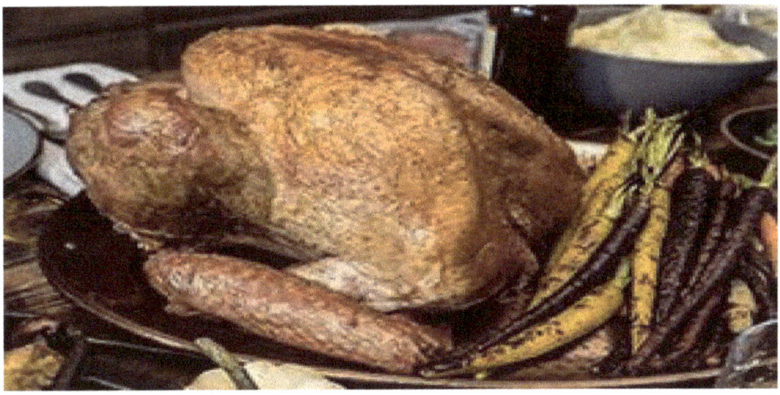

PREP TIME

15 MINS

COOK TIME

3 HRS

SERVES

4-6

HARDWOOD

APPLE

INGREDIENTS

TRAEGER ORANGE BRINE (FROM KIT)

TRAEGER TURKEY RUB (FROM KIT)

1.25-2.5 GALLONS COLD WATER

1 CUP BOURBON

1 TBSP. BUTTER, MELTED

1 TBSP. GRAND MARNIER OR OTHER ORANGE-FLAVORED LIQUOR

PREPARATION

Mix Traeger Orange Brine seasoning (from Orange Brine & Turkey Rub Kit) with one quart of water. Boil for 5 minutes. Remove from heat, add 1 gallon of cold water and bourbon. Refrigerate until completely cooled.

Place turkey breast side down in a large container. Pour cooled brine mix over bird. Add cold water until bird is submerged. Refrigerate for 24 hours.

Remove turkey and disregard brine. Blot turkey dry with paper towels. Combine butter and Grand Marnier and coat outside of turkey.

Season outside of turkey with Traeger Turkey Rub (from Orange Brine & Turkey Rub Kit).

When ready to cook, set temperature to 225°F and preheat, lid closed for 15 minutes.

Smoke turkey, breast up, for 2 hours. Increase temperature to 350°F and roast turkey until the internal temperature of the thickest part of the high reaches 165F, 2 to 3 hours, depending on size of turkey.

Let rest 20 to 30 minutes before serving. Enjoy!

HERB ROASTED TURKEY

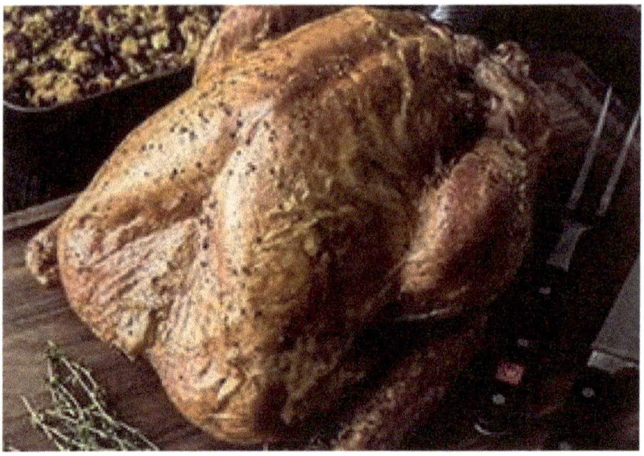

PREP TIME

15 MINS

COOK TIME

3 HRS

SERVES

6-8

HARDWOOD

HICKORY

INGREDIENTS

8 TBSP. BUTTER, ROOM TEMPERATURE

2 TBSP. MIXED HERBS SUCH AS PARSLEY, SAGE, ROSEMARY, AND MARJORAM, CHOPPED

1/4 TSP. BLACK PEPPER, FRESHLY GROUND

1 (12-14 LBS.) TURKEY, THAWED IF PREVIOUSLY FROZEN

3 TBSP. BUTTER

AS NEEDED TRAEGER PORK AND POULTRY RUB

2 CUPS CHICKEN OR TURKEY BROTH

PREPARATION

In a small mixing bowl, combine the 8 tablespoons of softened butter, mixed herbs, and black pepper and beat until fluffy with a wooden spoon. (You can make the herbed butter several days ahead: Cover and refrigerate, but bring to room temperature before using).

Remove any giblets from the turkey cavity and save them for gravy making, if desired. Wash the turkey, inside and out, under cold running water. Dry with paper towels. Place the turkey on a roasting rack in a roasting pan. Tuck the wings behind the back, and tie the legs together with butcher's string.

Using your fingers or the handle of a wooden spoon, gently push some of the herbed butter underneath the turkey skin onto the breast halves, being careful not to tear the skin. Massage the skin to evenly distribute the herbed butter.

Rub the outside of the turkey with the melted butter and sprinkle with the Traeger Pork and Poultry Rub. Pour the chicken broth in the bottom of the roasting pan.

When ready to cook, set temperature to 325°F and preheat, lid closed for 15 minutes.

Put the roasting pan with the turkey directly on the grill grate. Roast the turkey for 3 hours. Insert the probe from the meat thermometer in the thickest part of the thigh, but not touching bone. Cook until internal temperature reaches 165°F. The turkey should also be beautifully browned with crisp skin. If the temperature is less than that, or if your turkey is not browned to your liking, let it roast for another 30 minutes, then check the temperature again. Repeat until the turkey is fully cooked.

When the turkey is done, carefully transfer it to a cutting board and let it rest for 20 to 30 minutes. Do not tent it with aluminum foil or the skin will lose its crispness. Use the drippings that have accumulated in the bottom of the roasting pan to make gravy, if desired. Carve the turkey and serve.

TRAEGER LEFTOVER TURKEY SOUP

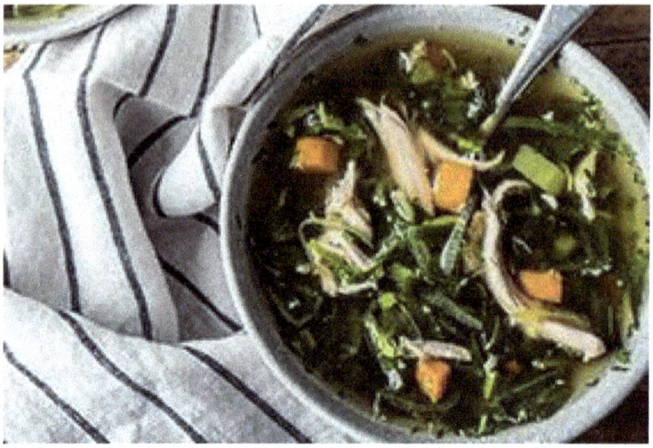

PREP TIME

15 MINS

COOK TIME

3 HRS

SERVES

4-6

HARDWOOD

APPLE

INGREDIENTS

1 TURKEY CARCASS

16 CUPS COLD WATER

2 LARGE CELERY RIBS, SLICED

2 LARGE CARROTS, SCRAPED AND SLICED

2 RED ONIONS, QUARTERED

10 SPRIGS FRESH FLAT PARSLEY LEAF

1 TBSP. PEPPERCORN

2 TSP. FRESH THYME

PREPARATION

Strip a turkey carcass of all meat; set aside in a container.

Break up the bones of the turkey carcass and place them in a large pot. Add any turkey skin or other assorted "bits" that are not edible meat. For the best taste, make the stock the day after the turkey has been cooked. Pour in the cold water and turn heat to high; bring to a boil.

Once the stock has come to a boil, add all remaining ingredients and turn heat down until the bubbles barely break the surface. Let simmer for 3 to 4 hours, stirring occasionally. The broth tastes best when reduced to 7 or 8 cups of stock.

When the stock is ready, strain it through a fine-meshed sieve into a large bowl; if your sieve is not fine, line it first with cheesecloth. Discard the bones and veggies you used to make the stock (all their flavor is now in the stock).

Refrigerate stock, covered, for several hours or preferably overnight. You can either make soup the next day, or freeze the stock; make sure you skim off the solidified fat before you either make soup or freeze the stock.

When ready to make the actual soup, heat up the homemade stock on the stovetop. Dish stock into individual bowls. Add shredded turkey, desired vegetables (such as chopped celery and red onions), fresh herbs (such as rosemary and thyme) and freshly ground pepper.

*Cook times will vary depending on set and ambient temperatures.

SMOKED TURKEY

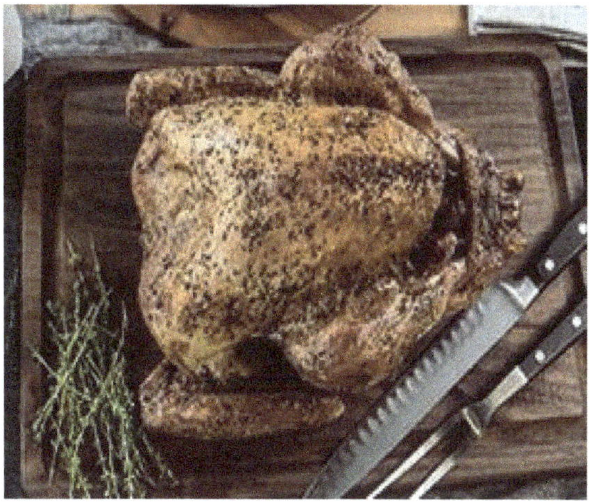

PREP TIME

8 HRS

COOK TIME

5 HRS

SERVES

6-8

HARDWOOD

HICKORY

INGREDIENTS

1 (12-14 LB) TURKEY, FRESH OR THAWED

3/4 LB (3 STICKS) UNSALTED BUTTER

1 (5 GAL) BUCKET OR STOCK POT

FOIL PAN, LARGE ENOUGH FOR TURKEY

HEAVY DUTY FOIL

BRINE

2 CUPS KOSHER SALT

2 CUPS SUGAR

2 GALS (1/2 GAL IS ICE) WATER

RUB

1/2 CUP KOSHER SALT

1/2 CUP COARSE GROUND BLACK PEPPER

PREPARATION

This method requires an overnight brining so collect everything the day before your meal.

The afternoon before, prepare your brine by adding the kosher salt and sugar to a medium saucepan. Cover with water and bring to a boil. Stir to dissolve the salt and sugar. Pour salt and sugar concentrate into a bucket, add ice and water up to 2 gallons.

Prepare your turkey by removing the neck, gizzards and truss, if pre-trussed. Trim off excess skin and fat near the cavity and neck. Place the turkey in bucket with the brine. If it floats, place a plate or two on top to keep the turkey submerged. Cover bucket and place in fridge until ready to cook the next afternoon.

When ready to cook, set temperature to 180°F and preheat, lid closed for 15 minutes.

Remove your turkey from the brine. Remember there's a cavity full of water so make sure to do this over the sink, otherwise you'll have brine all over the place. Set your turkey down on a cookie sheet to prepare it for the smoker.

Mix up the kosher salt and pepper in a shaker, sprinkle the rub on all parts of the turkey, don't sprinkle inside the cavity! There is no need to tie up the legs and wings with this method. The fan in the Traeger pushes air all around the turkey during the cook.

Put the turkey on the grill at 180°F for 2 hours, 225°F for the next hour, and finally 325°F to finish it off. Place it so the legs and thighs are towards the hotter area of your smoker and the breast to the cooler side. Check the turkey after a couple hours for color. When it reaches your desired color place it in the foil pan.

Cut the butter up into squares and pile them on the turkey.

Wrap in heavy-duty foil and put it back on the smoker. Cook until temperature in the breast reaches 165°F and the thigh reaches 180°F.

Remove from smoker and allow it to rest for 30 minutes before carving.

SMOKED TURKEY LEGS

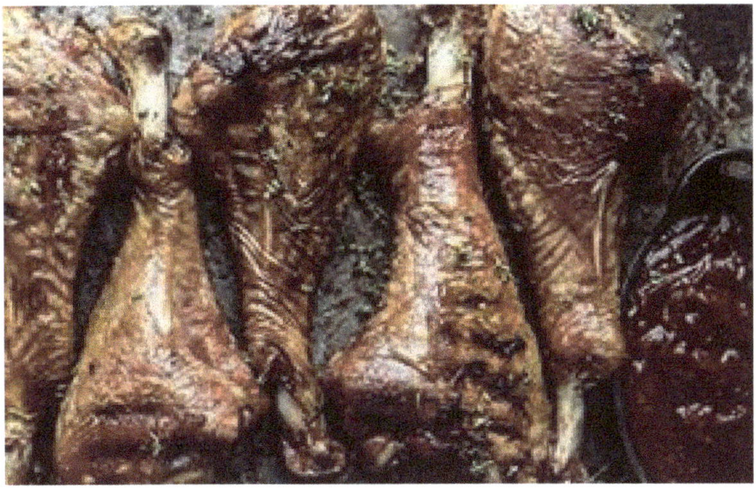

PREP TIME

24 HRS

COOK TIME

4-5 HRS

SERVES

4-6

HARDWOOD

HICKORY

INGREDIENTS

1 GAL WARM WATER

1/2 GAL COLD WATER

4 CUPS ICE

1 CUP TRAEGER BBQ RUB

1/2 CUP CURING SALT

1/2 CUP BROWN SUGAR

1 TBSP ALLSPICE BERRIES, CRUSHED (OPTIONAL)

1 TBSP WHOLE BLACK PEPPERCORNS

2 BAY LEAVES

2 TSP LIQUID SMOKE

4 TURKEY LEGS

PREPARATION

In a large stockpot, combine one gallon of warm water, the rub, curing salt, brown sugar, allspice (if using), peppercorns, bay leaves and liquid smoke.

Bring to a boil over high heat to dissolve the salt granules. Cool to room temperature.

Add cold water and ice; chill in the refrigerator. Add the turkey legs, making sure they're completely submerged in the brine.

After 24 hours, drain the turkey legs and discard the brine. Rinse the brine off the legs with cold water, then dry thoroughly with paper towels. Brush off any clinging solid spices.

When ready to cook, set temperature to 250°F and preheat, lid closed for 15 minutes.

Lay the turkey legs directly on the grill grate. Smoke for 4-5 hours, or until the internal temperature reaches 165°F on an instant-read meat thermometer. Make sure the probe doesn't touch bone or you'll get a false reading.

The turkey legs should be deeply browned. Don't be alarmed if the meat under the skin is pinkish: That's a chemical reaction to the cure and the smoke.

Serve immediately. Enjoy!

SMOKED TURKEY

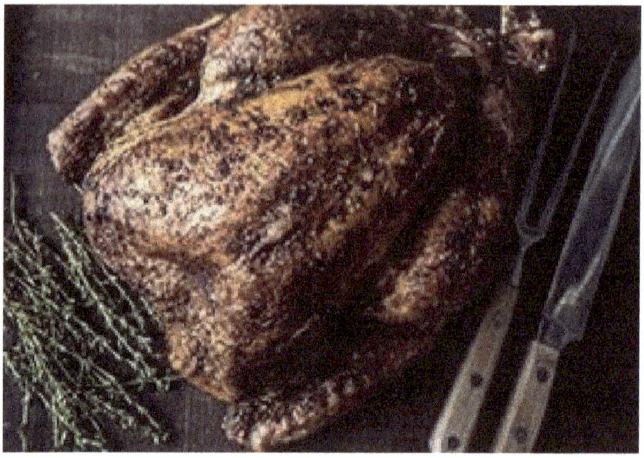

PREP TIME

24 HRS

COOK TIME

7 HRS

SERVES

6-8

HARDWOOD

PECAN

INGREDIENTS

1 (12-16 LB) FRESH OR FROZEN TURKEY, THAWED, ALL GIBLETS REMOVED

3 GAL WATER

1 CUP TRAEGER RUB

1 CUP SUGAR

1 1/2 TBSP GARLIC, MINCED

1/2 CUP WORCESTERSHIRE SAUCE

2 TBSP CANOLA OIL

PREPARATION

Ensure the turkey is fully thawed and remove any giblets.

Pour 3 gallons of water in a 5 gallon non-metal bucket. Add Traeger rub and mix until completely dissolved. Next add garlic, sugar, and Worcestershire sauce.

Place the turkey, breast side down, into the bucket with the brine. Make sure the turkey is completely submerged. Cover bucket and place in refrigerator overnight.

Remove turkey from brine and pat dry. Rub canola oil over entire outside of turkey and place breast side up into disposable aluminum roasting pan.

When ready to cook, set temperature to 225°F and preheat, lid closed for 15 minutes.

Place the turkey on the grill and smoke for 2 1/2 to 3 hours.

Increase grill temperature to 350°F and cook for 3-1/2 to 4 hours, or until the internal temperature reaches 165°F in the thickest part of the breast.

Remove from grill and allow to rest for 15 minutes before carving. Enjoy!

TRADITIONAL THANKSGIVING TURKEY

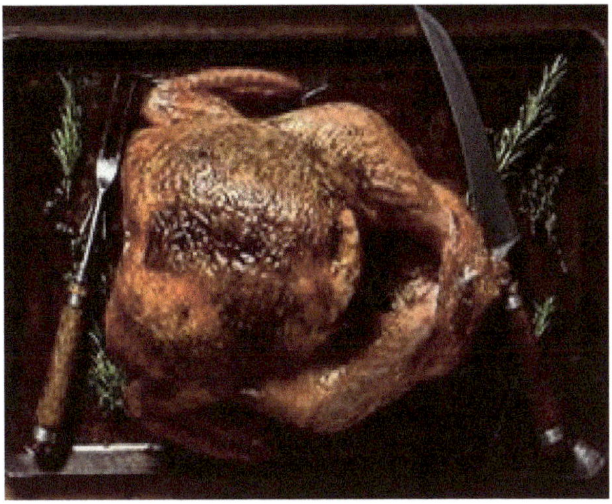

PREP TIME

15 MINS

COOK TIME

4 HRS

SERVES

8-12

HARDWOOD

CHERRY

INGREDIENTS

1 (18-20LB) TURKEY

1/2 LB BUTTER, SOFTENED

8 SPRIGS THYME

6 CLOVES GARLIC, MINCED

1 SPRIG ROSEMARY, ROUGH CHOP

1 TBSP CRACKED BLACK PEPPER

1/2 TBSP KOSHER SALT

PREPARATION

In a small bowl, combine butter with the minced garlic, thyme leaves, chopped rosemary, black pepper and kosher salt.

Prepare the turkey by separating the skin from the breast creating a pocket to stuff the butter-herb mixture in.

Cover the entire breast with 1/4" thickness of butter mixture.

Season the whole turkey with kosher salt and black pepper. As an option, you can also stuff the turkey cavity with Traditional Stuffing.

When ready to cook, set the temperature to 300°F and preheat, lid closed for 15 minutes.

Place turkey on the grill and roast for 3-4 hours. Check the internal temperature, the desired temperature is 175°F in the thigh next to the bone, and 160°F in the breast.

Turkey will continue to cook once taken off grill to reach a final temperature of 165°F in the breast.

Let rest for 10-15 minutes before carving. Enjoy!

HELLFIRE CHICKEN WINGS

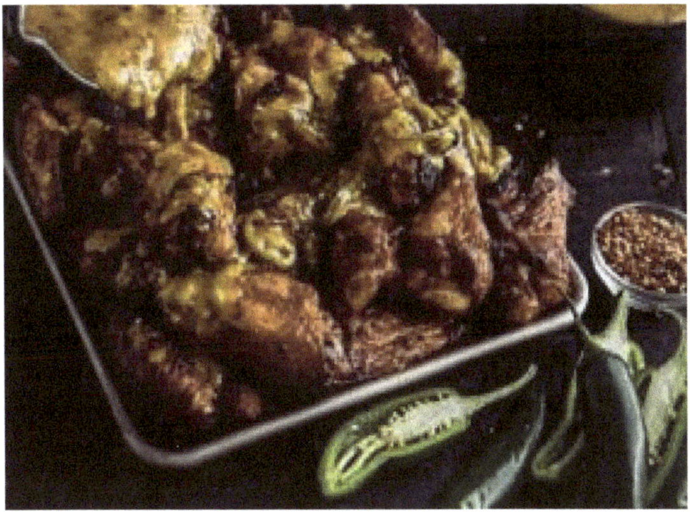

PREP TIME

15 MINS

COOK TIME

40 MINS

SERVES

4-6

HARDWOOD

HICKORY

INGREDIENTS

3 LBS. CHICKEN WINGS

2 TBSP. VEGETABLE OIL

RUB

1 TBSP. PAPRIKA

2 TSP. BROWN SUGAR

1 TSP. SALT

1 TSP. BLACK PEPPER, FRESHLY GROUND

1 TSP. CAYENNE PEPPER

1 TSP. ONION POWDER

1 TSP. GRANULATED GARLIC

1 TSP. CELERY SEED

SAUCE

8 TBSP. BUTTER, UNSALTED

2 - 4 JALAPENO PEPPERS, THINLY SLICED CROSSWISE

1/2 CUP CILANTRO LEAVES

1/2 CUP HOT SAUCE

PREPARATION

Cut the tips off wings and discard. Cut each wing into two pieces through the joint, giving you a meaty “drumette” and a “flat”. Transfer to a large mixing bowl and pour the oil over the chicken

Make the rub: In a small mixing bowl, combine the paprika, sugar, salt, black pepper, cayenne, onion powder, granulated garlic, and celery seed.

Sprinkle over the chicken and toss gently with your hands to coat the wings.

When ready to cook, set the temperature to 350°F and preheat, lid closed for 15 minutes

Grill the wings for 35 to 40 minutes, or until the skin is crisp and golden brown and the chicken is cooked through, turning once halfway through the cooking time.

Make the sauce: Melt the butter over medium-low heat in a small saucepan. Add the jalapeños and cook for 3-4 minutes. Stir in the cilantro & hot sauce.

Pour the sauce over the wings and toss to coat. Enjoy!

TURKEY JALAPENO MEATBALLS

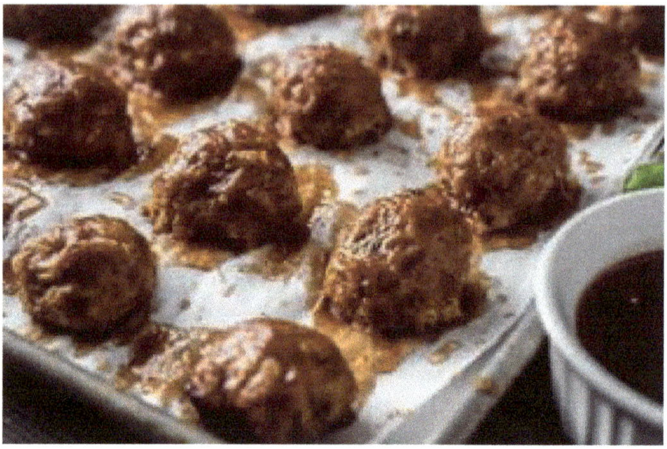

PREP TIME

15 MINS

COOK TIME

20 MINS

SERVES

8-12

HARDWOOD

HICKORY

INGREDIENTS

TURKEY JALAPEÑO MEATBALLS

1 1/4 LBS GROUND TURKEY

1 JALAPEÑO PEPPER, DESEEDED AND FINELY DICED

1/2 TSP GARLIC SALT

1 TSP ONION POWDER

1 TSP SALT

1/2 TSP GROUND BLACK PEPPER

1/4 TSP WORCESTERSHIRE SAUCE

CAYENNE PEPPER, PINCH

1 LARGE EGG, BEATEN

1/4 CUP MILK

1/2 CUP PLAIN BREAD CRUMBS OR PANKO

GLAZE

1 CUP CANNED JELLIED CRANBERRY SAUCE

1/2 CUP ORANGE MARMALADE

1/2 CUP CHICKEN BROTH

1 TBSP JALAPEÑO PEPPER, MINCED

SALT, TO TASTE

GROUND BLACK PEPPER, TO TASTE

PREPARATION

In a separate small bowl, combine the milk and bread crumbs.

In a large bowl, mix together turkey, garlic salt, onion powder, salt, pepper, Worcestershire sauce, cayenne pepper, egg and jalapeños.

Add the bread crumb milk mixture to the bowl and combine. Cover with plastic and refrigerate for up to 1 hour.

When ready to cook, set the temperature to 350°F and preheat, lid closed for 15 minutes

Roll the turkey mixture into balls, about one tablespoon each and place the meatballs in a single layer on a parchment lined baking sheet.

Cook meatballs until they start to brown, flipping occasionally until they reach an internal temperature of 175 degrees F and all sides are browned (about 20 minutes).

Glaze: Combine cranberry sauce, marmalade, chicken broth, and jalapeños and cook over medium heat in a small saucepan on the stovetop. Cook until ingredients are incorporated.

Half way through meatball cook time, brush the meatballs with the cranberry glaze.

Transfer meatballs to a serving dish with cranberry glaze on the side. Serve immediately. Enjoy!

BUFFALO CHICKEN THIGHS

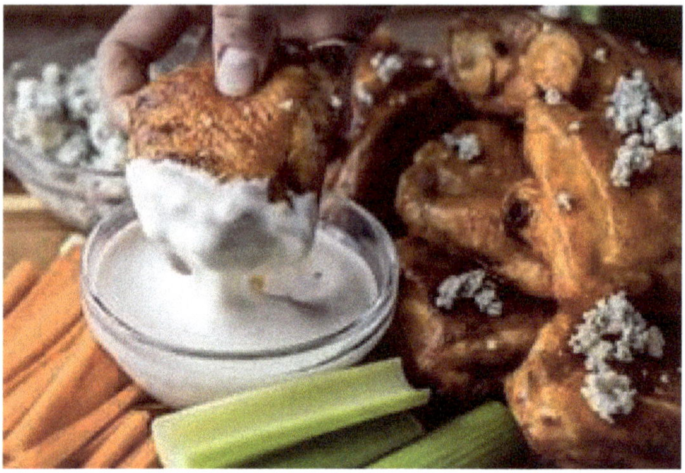

PREP TIME

5 MINS

COOK TIME

15 MINS

SERVES

4-6

HARDWOOD

MESQUITE

INGREDIENTS

4-6 BONELESS, SKINLESS CHICKEN THIGHS

1 CUP BUFFALO WING SAUCE

4 TBSP. BUTTER

TRAEGER PORK & POULTRY RUB, AS NEEDED

BLEU CHEESE CRUMBLES, FOR SERVING

RANCH DRESSING, FOR SERVING

PREPARATION

When ready to cook, set the temperature to 450°F and preheat, lid closed for 15 minutes.

Generously season the chicken thighs with your desired Traeger seasoning and place directly on the grill grate. Cook for 8-10 minutes, flipping once.

In a small saucepan, cook the wing sauce and the butter over medium heat stirring occasionally.

Dip the cooked chicken thighs into the wing sauce and butter mixture, turning to coat both sides evenly.

Return the sauced chicken thighs to the grill and cook for an additional 4-5 minutes or until the internal temperature reads 175 degrees on a meat thermometer.

Sprinkle with the Bleu cheese and drizzle with the ranch dressing (optional). We like to serve ours as sliders on toasted buns with all the fixings. Enjoy!

WILD TURKEY SOUTHWEST EGG ROLLS

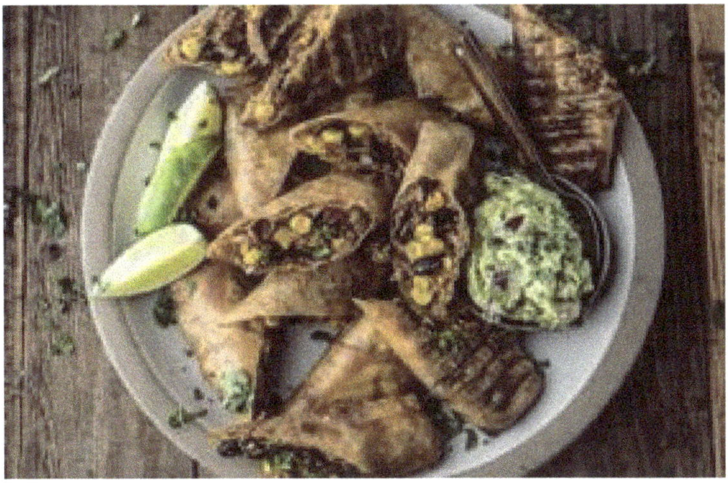

PREP TIME

15 MINS

COOK TIME

40 MINS

SERVES

4-6

HARDWOOD

TURKEY BLEND

INGREDIENTS

2 CUPS LEFTOVER WILD TURKEY MEAT

1/2 CUP CORN

1/2 CUP BLACK BEANS

3 TBSP TACO SEASONING

1/2 CUP WHITE ONION, CHOPPED

4 CLOVES GARLIC, MINCED

1 POBLANO PEPPER (OR 2 JAPALEÑO PEPPERS), CHOPPED

1 CAN ROTEL TOMATOES & CHILES

1/2 CUP WATER

12 EGG ROLL WRAPPERS

PREPARATION

Add olive oil to a large skillet and heat on the stove over medium heat. Add onions and peppers and sauté 2-3 minutes until soft. Add garlic, cook 30 seconds, then Rotel and black beans. Reduce heat and simmer.

Pour taco seasoning over meat and add 1/3 cup of water and mix to coat well. Add to veggie mixture and stir to mix well. If it seems dry, add 2 tbsp water. Cook until heated all the way through.

Remove from the heat and transfer the mixture to the fridge. The mixture should be completely cooled prior to stuffing the egg rolls or the wrappers will break.

Place spoonful of the mixture in each wrapper and wrap tightly. Repeat with remaining wrappers. When ready to cook, set temperature to High and preheat, lid closed for 15 minutes.

Brush each egg roll with oil or butter and place directly on the Traeger grill grate. Cook until the exterior is crispy, about 20 min per side.

Remove from Traeger and cool. Serve. Enjoy!

BEER BRAISED CHICKEN TACOS WITH JALAPEÑO RELISH

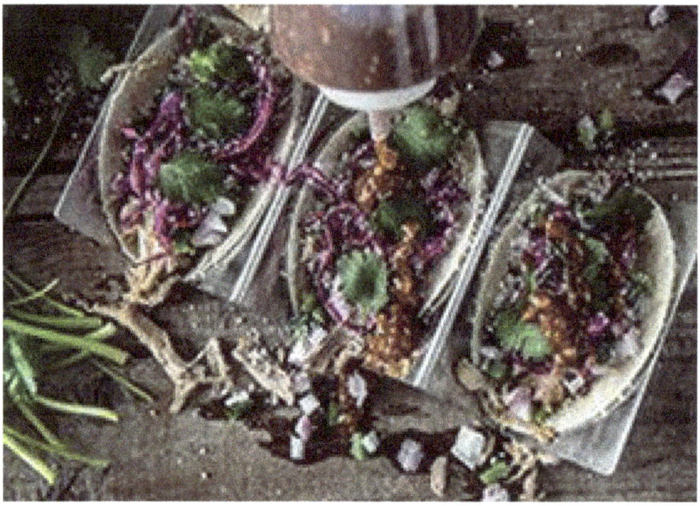

PREP TIME

20 MINS

COOK TIME

40 MINS

SERVES

8-12

HARDWOOD

PECAN

INGREDIENTS

JALAPEÑO RELISH

3 JALAPEÑOS, SEEDED AND DICED

1/4 CUP RED ONION, FINELY DICED

1 CLOVE GARLIC, MINCED

2/3 CUP WHITE WINE VINEGAR

1/3 CUP WATER

1 TBSP SUGAR

1 TBSP SALT

PICKLED CABBAGE

2 CUPS SHREDDED RED CABBAGE

1/2 CUP WHITE WINE VINEGAR

1 TBSP SALT

1 TBSP SUGAR

BRAISED CHICKEN

2 LBS BONELESS SKINLESS CHICKEN THIGHS

1 TBSP OLIVE OIL

1 TSP SALT

1 TSP BLACK PEPPER

1/2 YELLOW ONION, SMALL DICE

1 JALAPEÑO, DESEEDED AND CHOPPED

1 CLOVE GARLIC, MINCED

1 TSP CHILI POWDER

1 TSP GARLIC POWDER

4 TBSP ADOBO SAUCE

1 EA CHIPOTLE CHILE IN ADOBO

JUICE OF 2 LIMES

1 (12 OZ) CAN MODELO BEER

TACOS

8-12 SMALL FLOUR TORTILLAS

COTIJA CHEESE

CILANTRO

YOUR FAVORITE HOT SAUCE

PREPARATION

For the jalapeño relish, combine all ingredients in a non-reactive dish and set aside.

To make the pickled cabbage, combine all ingredients in a non-reactive dish and set aside.

Transfer both the relish and pickled cabbage to the refrigerator and let sit a couple hours to overnight.

Season chicken thighs generously with salt and pepper. Heat 1 Tbsp olive oil in a dutch oven over medium-high heat. Place chicken thighs skin side down and brown in batches. Remove from heat and set aside.

Add 1 Tbsp butter to the dutch oven and set over medium-high heat. When butter is melted, add onion and jalapeño and sauté 3-5 minutes until translucent. Add minced garlic and sauté 30 seconds or until fragrant.

Add chili powder, adobo sauce, chipotle Chile and lime juice. Add chicken thighs back to the dutch oven and pour in beer.

When ready to cook, set the Traeger to 350°F and preheat, lid closed for 15 minutes.

Place dutch oven in the grill and braise for 30 minutes or until chicken is tender and falls apart. Remove chicken from braising liquid and shred.

To build the tacos, place shredded chicken on tortilla, top with jalapeño relish, cabbage, cotija, cilantro, and finish with hot sauce. Enjoy!

SLOW ROASTED SHAWARMA

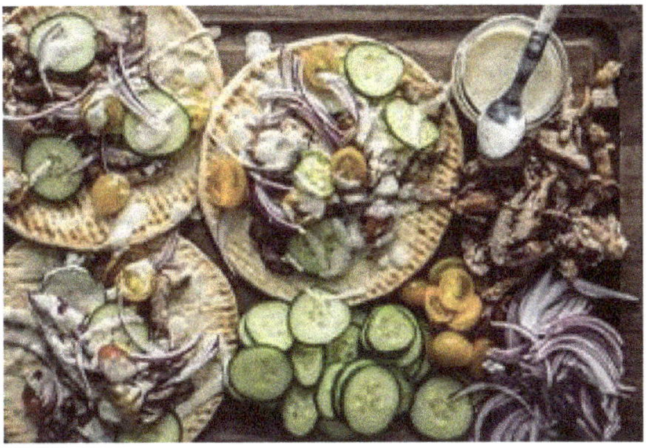

PREP TIME

25 MINS

COOK TIME

4.5 HRS

SERVES

6-8

HARDWOOD

MESQUITE

INGREDIENTS

5.5 LBS TOP SIRLOIN

5.5 LBS BONELESS SKINLESS CHICKEN THIGHS

4.5 LBS LAMB FAT

4 TBSP TRAEGER RUB

2 LARGE YELLOW ONIONS

PITA BREAD

TOPPING OPTIONS: CUCUMBER, TOMATOES, TAHINI, PICKLES, FRIES, ISRAELI SALAD

A DOUBLE SKEWER

A CAST IRON GRIDDLE

PREPARATION

*Plan ahead! Assemble the shawarma stack the night before you plan to cook it.

Slice all the meat and fat into ½" slices and place into 3 bowls (pro tip: it's easier to slice if they are all partially frozen).

Season each bowl with Traeger Rub and massage the rub into the meat.

Place half an onion on the bottom of each half skewer to make a firm base. then add 2 layers from each bowl at a time. Try to make the stack symmetrical, more or less. Then put the other 2 half onions at the top. Wrap in plastic wrap and refrigerate overnight.

When ready to cook, set temperature to 275°F and preheat, lid closed for 15 minutes.

Lay the shawarma directly on the grill grate and cook for about 3-4 hours, rotating at least once.

Remove from grill and increase the temperature to 445°F. While the grill preheats, place a cast iron griddle directly on the grill grate and brush with olive oil.

When the griddle is hot place the whole shawarma on the cast iron and sear 5-10 minutes per side. Remove from grill, slice off the edges, then repeat with remaining shawarma.

Serve in pita bread with your favorite toppings like cucumber, tomatoes, tahini, pickles, fries or Israeli salad.

Enjoy!

BBQ CHICKEN NACHOS

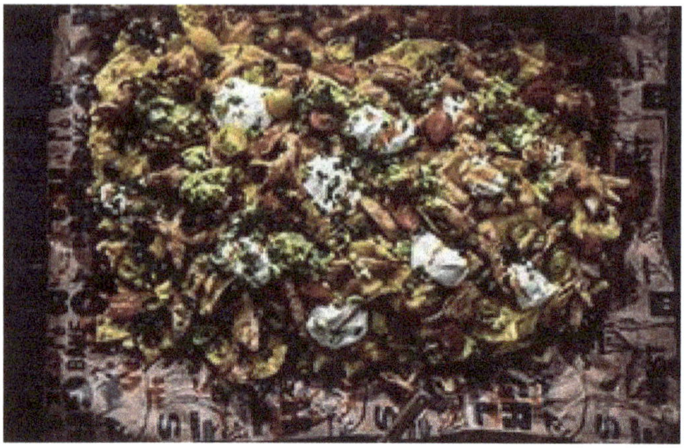

PREP TIME

10 MINS

COOK TIME

45 MINS

SERVES

4-6

HARDWOOD

MAPLE

INGREDIENTS

1-1/4 LBS. CHICKEN BREASTS, BONELESS, SKINLESS

TRAEGER PORK & POULTRY RUB, AS NEEDED

1/2 TO 3/4 CUP TRAEGER 'QUE BBQ SAUCE

24 LARGE TORTILLA CHIPS

3 CUPS MEXICAN BLEND SHREDDED CHEESE

1/2 CUP BLACK OLIVES, SLICED AND DRAINED

PICKLED JALAPENOS, SLICED

3 SCALLIONS, THINLY SLICED

1 CUP SOUR CREAM

PREPARATION

Season the chicken breasts with the Traeger Pork and Poultry Rub.

When ready to cook, set temperature to 350°F and preheat, lid closed for 15 minutes.

Arrange the chicken breasts on the grill grate and cook, turning once halfway through the cooking time, for 25 to 30 minutes, or until the internal temperature when read on an instant-read meat thermometer is 170°F. Transfer to a cutting board and let rest for 3 minutes. Leave the grill on if you are making the nachos immediately.

Dice the chicken into small cubes, 1/2-inch or less. Transfer to a mixing bowl and pour 1/2 cup of Traeger Regular Barbecue Sauce over the diced chicken. Stir gently to coat each piece.

Set aside, or cover and refrigerate if not making the nachos immediately. Lay the tortilla chips in a single layer on a rimmed baking sheet or pizza pan. Sprinkle evenly with half the cheese and a few of the jalepenos (if using).

Spoon barbecued chicken mixture on each chip. Top with black olives and more pickled jalapeno, if desired. Sprinkle the remaining half of the cheese evenly over the chips. Scatter the sliced onions over the chips.

Put the baking sheet on the grill grate. Bake until the chips are crisp and the cheese is melted, 12 to 15 minutes. With a spatula, transfer the nachos to a plate or platter. Serve immediately with sou cream and pickled jalepenos. Enjoy!

SPICY BBQ CHICKEN

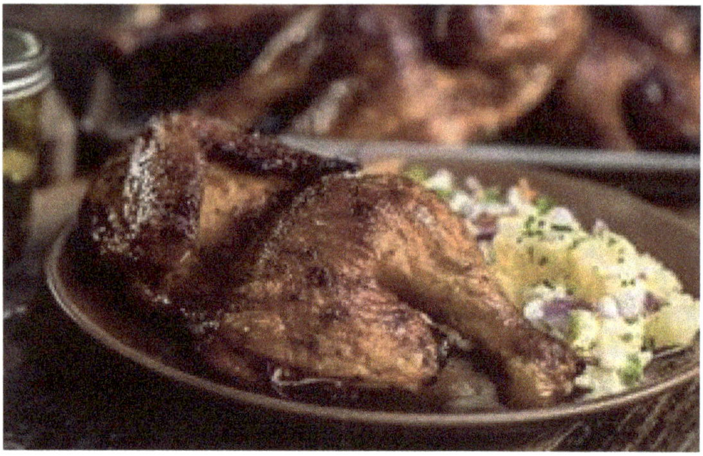

PREP TIME

30 MINS

COOK TIME

60 MINS

SERVES

2-4

HARDWOOD

APPLE

INGREDIENTS

1 WHOLE CHICKEN

6 THAI CHILES

2 TBSP SWEET PAPRIKA

1 SCOTCH BONNET

2 TBSP SUGAR

3 TBSP SALT

1 WHITE ONION

5 GARLIC CLOVES

4 CUPS GRAPE SEED OIL

PREPARATION

Puree the thai chilies, paprika, scotch bonnet, sugar, salt, onion, garlic, and grape seed oil together until smooth.

Smother the chicken with mixture and let rest in fridge overnight.

When ready to cook, set the Traeger to 300°F and preheat, lid closed for 15 minutes.

Place chicken on grill breast side up and smoke for 3 hours or until it reaches an internal temperature of 165°F in the breast.

Remove from grill and allow to rest for 10 to 15 minutes before slicing.

Serve with sides of choice. Enjoy!

TRAEGER BBQ HALF CHICKENS

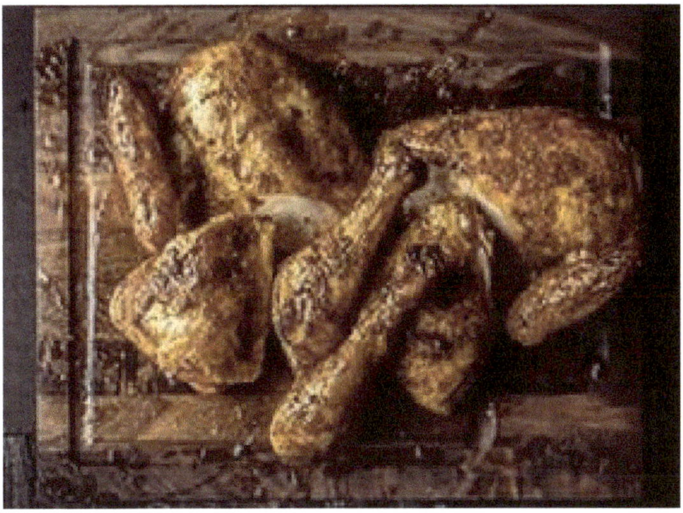

PREP TIME

15 MINS

COOK TIME

75 MINS

SERVES

2-4

HARDWOOD

APPLE

INGREDIENTS

1 EA (3-3 1/2 LB) YOUNG FRESH CHICKEN

TRAEGER APRICOT BBQ SAUCE

TRAEGER SUMMER SHANDY RUB

PREPARATION

Place the chicken, breast side down, on a cutting board with the neck pointing away from you. Cut along one side of the backbone, staying as close to the bone as possible, from the neck to the tail.

Repeat on the other side of the backbone then remove it. Open the chicken and slice through the white cartilage at the tip of the breastbone to pop it open. Cut down either side of the breast bone then use your fingers to pull it out.

Flip the chicken over so it is skin side up and cut down the center splitting the chicken in half. Tuck the wings back of each chicken half.

Season on both sides with Traeger Summer Shandy rub.

When ready to cook, set the temperature to 375°F and preheat, lid closed for 15 minutes.

Place chicken directly on the grill grate skin side up and cook until the internal temperature reaches 160 degrees F, about 60-90 minutes.

Brush the BBQ sauce all over the chicken skin and cook for an additional 10 minutes.

Remove from grill and let rest 5 minutes before serving. Enjoy!

EGGS

SMOKED DEVILED EGGS

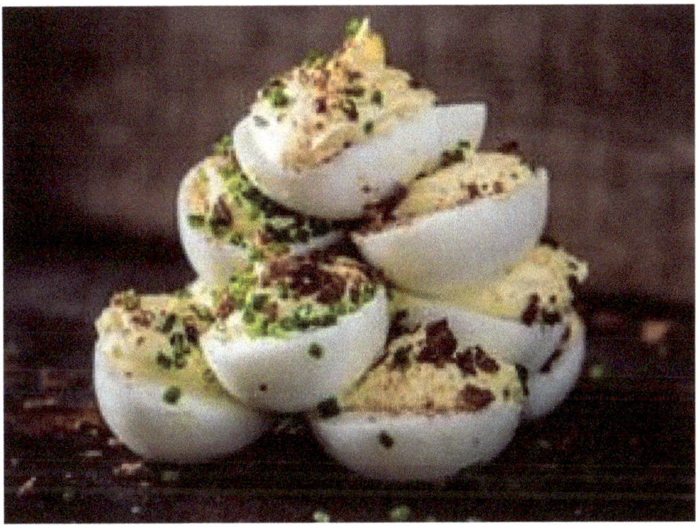

PREP TIME

15 MINS

COOK TIME

30 MINS

SERVES

4-6

HARDWOOD

HICKORY

INGREDIENTS

7 HARD BOILED EGGS, COOKED AND PEELED

3 TBSP MAYONNAISE

3 TSP CHIVES, DICED

1 TSP BROWN MUSTARD

1 TSP APPLE CIDER VINEGAR

DASH OF HOT SAUCE

SALT AND PEPPER, TO TASTE

2 TBSP BACON, CRUMBLED

PAPRIKA, FOR DUSTING

PREPARATION

When ready to cook, set temperature to 180°F and preheat, lid closed for 15 minutes. For optimal flavor, use Super Smoke if available.

Place cooked and peeled eggs directly on the grill grate and smoke eggs for 30 minutes. Remove from grill and allow eggs to cool.

Slice the eggs lengthwise and scoop the egg yolks into a gallon zip top bag. Add mayonnaise, chives, mustard, vinegar, hot sauce, salt, and pepper to the bag.

Zip the bag closed and, using your hands, knead all of the ingredients together until completely smooth.

Squeeze the yolk mixture into one corner of the bag and cut a small part of the corner off. Pipe the yolk mixture into the hard boiled egg whites.

Top the deviled eggs with crumbled bacon and paprika. Chill until ready to serve. Enjoy!

SANDWICH

PICKLED BRINED HOT CHICKEN SANDWICH

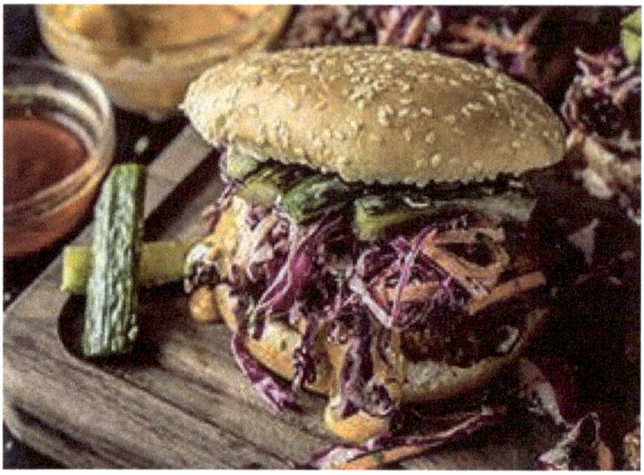

PREP TIME

20 MINS

COOK TIME

25 MINS

SERVES

8-12

HARDWOOD

APPLE

INGREDIENTS

PICKLE BRINED CHICKEN

2 CUPS LEFTOVER PICKLE JUICE

8 EA BONELESS SKINLESS CHICKEN THIGHS

SALT AND PEPPER, AS NEEDED

1 CUP FLOUR

1/2 CUP TAPIOCA FLOUR

1 CUP BUTTERMILK

2 TSP FRANKS RED HOT SAUCE

1 EGG

BUTTER HOT SAUCE

1/2 CUP BUTTER, MELTED

1/2 CUP FRANKS RED HOT SAUCE

2 TSP CAYENNE

1/2 TSP DARK BROWN SUGAR

1 TSP BLACK PEPPER

1 TSP GARLIC

1 TSP PAPRIKA

SANDWICH

SHREDDED CABBAGE SLAW

TRAEGER SMOKED PICKLES

4 SESAME SEED BUNS

PREPARATION

In a medium bowl, combine pickle juice and chicken thighs. Weigh them down if necessary to make sure they are completely submerged. Place in the refrigerator to brine overnight.

When ready to cook, set the temperature to High and preheat, lid closed for 15 minutes.

Place a cast iron pan with 1/2-inch canola oil on the grill grate while the grill preheats.

Remove the chicken thighs from the pickle brine and pat dry.

In a medium bowl combine both flours and a pinch of salt. Mix well to combine.

In another bowl combine the buttermilk, hot sauce, egg and a pinch of salt. Mix well to combine.

Season the chicken thighs with salt. Dip the thighs in the flour mixture, then buttermilk, then back into the flour mixture. Transfer to a wire rack and repeat with the remaining thighs.

Place wire rack directly on the grill grate next to the cast iron of oil and bake chicken for 15 minutes or until the internal temperature reaches 150°F.

As chicken pieces come to temperature, transfer them 2 or 3 at a time to the preheated oil to crisp the coating and finish cooking.

For the Butter Hot Sauce: While the chicken is cooking, melt the butter and combine with the hot sauce, brown sugar, cayenne, garlic powder, paprika and black pepper in a medium bowl. Set aside.

Remove chicken from the oil when the internal temperature reaches 165°F and dunk in the butter hot sauce mixture.

Build the sandwiches with buns, mayonnaise, pickles, cabbage slaw and hot chicken. Enjoy!

CHICKEN CORDON BLEU

BAKED CHICKEN CORDON BLEU

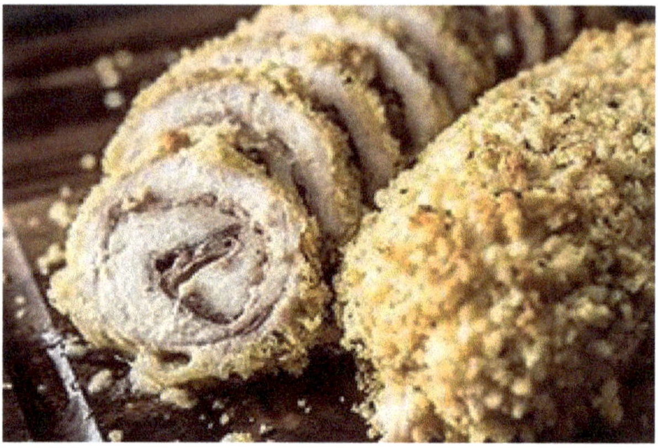

PREP TIME

90 MINS

COOK TIME

30 MINS

SERVES

4-6

HARDWOOD

ALDER

INGREDIENTS

4 EA (4-5 OZ) BONELESS, SKINLESS CHICKEN BREASTS

8 SLICES PROSCIUTTO OR HAM

8 SLICES SWISS CHEESE

1/3 CUP ALL-PURPOSE FLOUR

SALT, AS NEEDED

FRESHLY GROUND BLACK PEPPER, AS NEEDED

1 CUP DRY BREADCRUMBS, PREFERABLY PANKO

1/4 CUP GRATED PARMESAN CHEESE

2 TBSP MELTED BUTTER

2 TSP FRESH THYME LEAVES

2 EGGS

PREPARATION

Spray a baking sheet with nonstick cooking spray. Set aside.

Butterfly each chicken breast and place between two pieces of plastic wrap. Evenly pound with the flat side of a meat mallet, being careful not to tear the chicken, until chicken is 1/4-inch thick.

Lay each chicken breast on a fresh piece of plastic wrap. Season chicken with salt and lay 1 to 2 slices of cheese on each breast followed by prosciutto or ham, then 1-2 more slices of cheese.

Roll the chicken breast up like you would roll a burrito. Using the bottom piece of plastic wrap as an aid, fold the bottom of the breast up about an inch, then fold in the sides. Roll tightly.

Wrap in the plastic wrap and tightly twist the ends to shape and compress the chicken. Repeat with the remaining chicken breasts. Chill in the refrigerator for 60 minutes.

While chicken chills, season the flour with salt and pepper and put in a shallow dish.

Combine the breadcrumbs, parmesan cheese, butter, and thyme. Season with salt and pepper and put in a second shallow dish.

Whisk the eggs in a separate third dish.

Arrange your workspace in this order: flour, eggs, breadcrumbs. Put the prepared baking sheet next to the breadcrumbs.

Remove the plastic wrap from the chicken breasts. Coat each lightly with flour then dip in the egg.

Finally, roll in breadcrumbs, patting them to make them adhere. Arrange on the baking sheet.

When ready to cook, set the temperature to 375°F and preheat, lid closed for 15 minutes.

Place the baking sheet with the chicken on the grill. Bake for 30-40 minutes, or until the coating is golden brown and the chicken is cooked through.

Serve whole or slice crosswise into pinwheels with a sharp serrated knife. Enjoy!

WINGS

ROASTED TERIYAKI WINGS

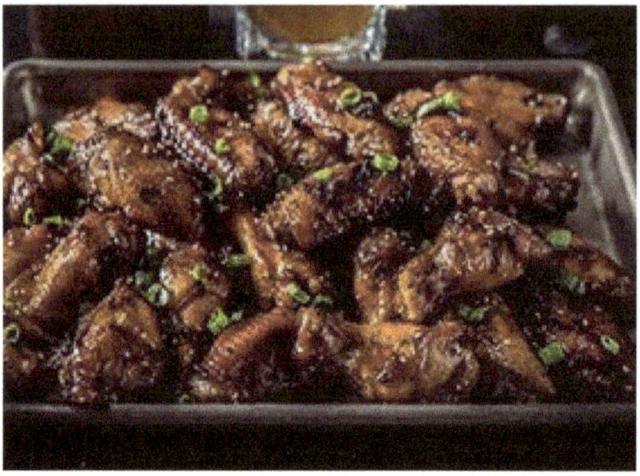

PREP TIME

4 HRS

COOK TIME

60 MINS

SERVES

6-8

HARDWOOD

MAPLE

INGREDIENTS

2 1/2 LBS LARGE CHICKEN WINGS

1/2 CUP SOY SAUCE

1/4 CUP WATER

1/4 CUP BROWN SUGAR

2 TBSP RICE WINE VINEGAR

2 SCALLIONS

1 CLOVE GARLIC, MINCED

2 TSP SESAME OIL

2 TBSP FRESH GINGER, SMASHED

1 TBSP SESAME SEEDS, LIGHTLY TOASTED

PREPARATION

Cut the wings into three pieces through the joints. Discard the wing tips, or save for chicken stock.

Transfer the remaining chicken drumettes and flats to a large resealable plastic bag or a bowl.

For the Marinade: In a small saucepan, combine the soy sauce, water, brown sugar, vinegar, scallions, garlic, sesame oil, and ginger. Bring to a boil, then reduce the heat and simmer for 10 minutes.

Cool completely, then pour over the chicken wings. Seal the bag and refrigerate for several hours, or overnight. Drain the wings, discarding the marinade.

When ready to cook, set the temperature to 350°F and preheat, lid closed for 15 minutes.

Cook for 45 to 50 minutes, or until the skin is brown and crisp and the meat is no longer pink at the bone.

Turn once during the cooking time to prevent the wings from sticking to the grill grate. Remove from grill.

Sprinkle with sesame seeds to serve. Enjoy!

SMOKED KOREAN WINGS

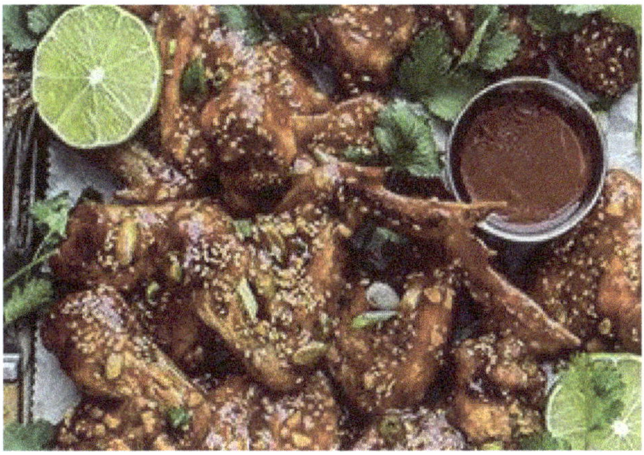

PREP TIME

3 HRS

COOK TIME

60 MINS

SERVES

4-6

HARDWOOD

CHERRY

INGREDIENTS

BRINE

1 GALLON WATER

1 CUP SEA SALT

1/2 CUP SUGAR

1 LEMON, HALVED

1 HEAD GARLIC, HALVED

4 SPRIGS THYME

10 PEPPERCORNS

WINGS

3 LB CHICKEN WINGS

2 TBSP OLIVE OIL

SAUCE

1/2 CUP GOCHUJANG HOT PEPPER PASTE#1

1/4 CUP SOY SAUCE

1/3 CUP HONEY

2 TBSP RICE WINE VINEGAR

2 TBSP FRESH SQUEEZED LIME JUICE

2 TBSP TOASTED SESAME OIL

1/4 CUP BUTTER, MELTED

4 CLOVES GARLIC, MINCED

1 TBSP GINGER, PEELED AND GRATED

PREPARATION

For the Brine: To a stockpot, add 1 gallon of water, salt, and sugar, and stir well. Bring to a boil then remove from the heat and stir in the lemon, garlic, thyme, and peppercorns. Cool to room temperature, then submerge the wings. Cover and refrigerate for 2 to 4 hours.

When ready to cook, set the temperature to 375°F and preheat, with the lid closed for 15 minutes.

Remove the wings from the brine and dry them completely with paper towel. Discard brine.

Toss the wings with the olive oil coating them completely.

Place the wings directly onto the grill grate and cook to an internal temperature of 165°F, about 45 to 60 minutes.

For the Sauce: In a bowl, combine all the sauce ingredients and whisk until smooth. Heat over medium-heat until the sauce just comes to a simmer, then remove from heat and set aside.

Toss the cooked wings with 2/3 of the sauce, the green onions, peanuts, and sesame seeds.

Serve wings with fresh cilantro, lime wedges, and extra sauce for dipping. Enjoy!

ROASTED BUFFALO WINGS

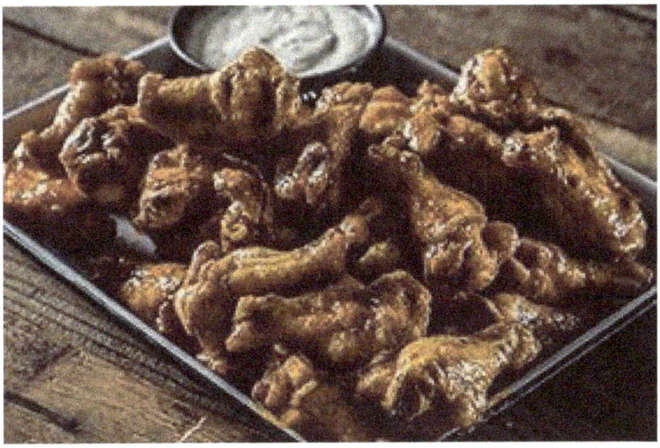

PREP TIME

10 MINS

COOK TIME

30 MINS

SERVES

4-6

HARDWOOD

HICKORY

INGREDIENTS

CHICKEN WINGS

4 LBS CHICKEN WINGS

1 TBSP CORN STARCH

TRAEGER CHICKEN RUB, AS NEEDED

KOSHER SALT, TO TASTE

BUFFALO SAUCE

1/4 CUP SPICY MUSTARD

1/2 CUP FRANKS RED HOT SAUCE

6 TBSP UNSALTED BUTTER

PREPARATION

When ready to cook, set the temperature to 375°F and preheat, lid closed for 15 minutes.

While grill is preheating, dry off chicken wings with a paper towel. Place wings in a large bowl and sprinkle with cornstarch, Traeger Chicken Rub and salt to taste. Mix to coat both sides of the chicken wings.

When the grill has heated, place the wings on the grill and cook for 35 minutes total, turning halfway through cook time.

Check the internal temperature of the wings at 35 minutes. The internal temperature should be at least

165°F. However, an internal temperature of 175-180°F will yield a better texture.

For the Buffalo Sauce: In another pot add the Franks Red Hot, mustard and butter. Whisk to combine and heat through on the stove top.

Keep sauce warm while the wings are cooking. When wings are done, pour the buffalo sauce over the wings, turning with tongs to coat.

Cook for an additional 10-15 minutes on the grill for the sauce to set.

Serve wings with ranch or blue cheese dressing. Enjoy!

ROASTED TEQUILA-LIME WINGS

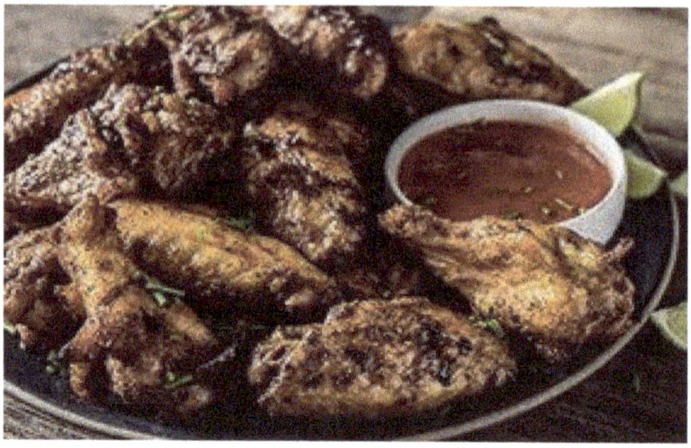

PREP TIME

15 MINS

COOK TIME

30 MINS

SERVES

6-8

HARDWOOD

HICKORY

INGREDIENTS

WINGS

3 LBS CHICKEN WINGS

2 TSP ANCHO CHILE POWDER

2 TSP BROWN SUGAR

1 TSP GRANULATED GARLIC

1 TSP CUMIN

1 TSP KOSHER SALT

1 TSP CHILI POWDER

2 TBSP VEGETABLE OIL

GLAZE

1/4 CUP HONEY

1/4 CUP PINEAPPLE JUICE

3 TBSP TEQUILA

1-1/2 TBSP HOT SAUCE

1-1/2 TBSP BUTTER

1-1/2 TBSP FRESH LIME JUICE

PREPARATION

When ready to cook, set temperature to High and preheat, lid closed for 15 minutes.

If you bought whole chicken wings, remove the tip and separate the drumettes and wings from each other. Pat them dry. Discard the wing tips or save them for chicken stock.

Combine all of the dry rub ingredients in a medium bowl. Add the oil and whisk to combine. Add the chicken wings and toss well to coat.

For the Glaze: Combine glaze ingredients in a small saucepan. Bring to a boil over medium heat. Cook until mixture is reduced by about 1/3 and begins to thicken, about 3 minutes. Keep the syrup warm while waiting to glaze.

Place the wings directly on the grill grate and cook, turning once, until the internal temperature of the wings reach 155-160°F, about 20 minutes.

Brush the wings with the glaze and continue to cook until the internal temperature reaches 165-175°F, about 5-10 minutes longer.

Serve warm. Enjoy!

SMOKED

SMOKED CHICKEN TIKKA MASALA

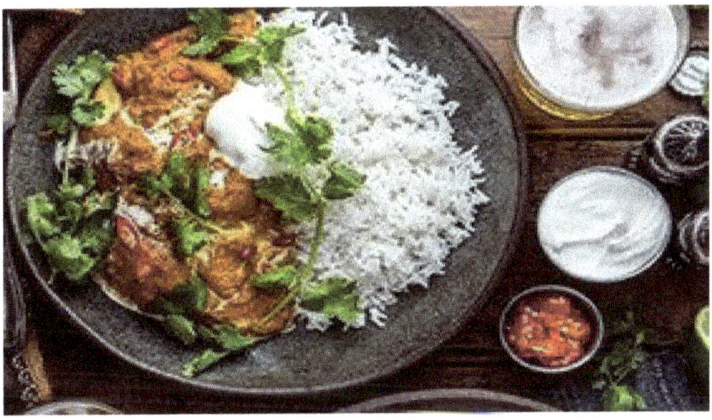

PREP TIME

30 MINS

COOK TIME

45 MINS

SERVES

4-6

HARDWOOD

MESQUITE

INGREDIENTS

MARINADE

6 GARLIC CLOVES, MINCED

1 THUMB-SIZED KNOB OF GINGER, FINELY DICED

4 TSP GROUND TURMERIC

2 TSP GARAM MASALA

2 TSP GROUND CORIANDER

2 TSP GROUND CUMIN

2 TSP GROUND CHILI

1 1/2 CUPS WHOLE MILK YOGHURT

1 TBSP KOSHER SALT

2 LB CHICKEN BREASTS, CUT INTO 1-INCH STRIPS

TIKKA MASALA SAUCE

3 TBSP GHEE OR CLARIFIED BUTTER

1 MEDIUM ONION, FINELY DICED

FINELY DICED CILANTRO STEMS 1/4 CUP

TOMATO PASTE 1/4 CUP

6 CARDAMOM PODS, CRUSHED

1 (28 OZ) CAN CRUSHED TOMATOES

2 CUPS HEAVY WHIPPING CREAM

1-2 SLICED FRESH CHILIES, FOR GARNISH

1/2 CUP FRESH CILANTRO, FOR GARNISH

1 CUP CREAMY YOGURT

COOKED BASMATI RICE, TO SERVE

PREPARATION

Prepare the spice mixture by combining the garlic, ginger and all the spices in a small bowl. Mix well and set aside.

For the Marinade: In a large bowl, combine the sliced chicken breast, yogurt, 1/2 the spice mixture, and kosher salt. Mix well.

Cover with plastic wrap and chill in the fridge overnight for marinated chicken perfection.

When ready to cook, set the temperature to High and preheat with the lid closed for 15 minutes.

For the Sauce: Heat a high-sided, oven-safe pan over medium-heat and melt the ghee. Add the onion, cilantro stems, cardamom, and a pinch of salt, and cook until the onion softens, about 5 minutes. Add the tomato paste and remaining spice mixture, and cook for 2 minutes. Pour in the tomatoes and season with another pinch of salt. Bring the sauce to a simmer and cook for about 8 minutes, until thickened.

While the sauce is cooking, add the marinated chicken pieces to the grill and cook for 2 minutes per side, until just starting to turn to beautifully golden brown. Remove and set aside.

Reduce grill heat to 350°F. Stir the cream into the sauce mixture, then fold in the chicken. Transfer the curry to the grill and cook, lid closed, for 35 to 40 minutes, until the chicken is cooked through and the curry is thick and glorious.

Divide the cooked basmati rice onto plates, then top with curry. Garnish with yogurt, fresh chilies and cilantro. Enjoy!

ROASTED ROSEMARY ORANGE CHICKEN

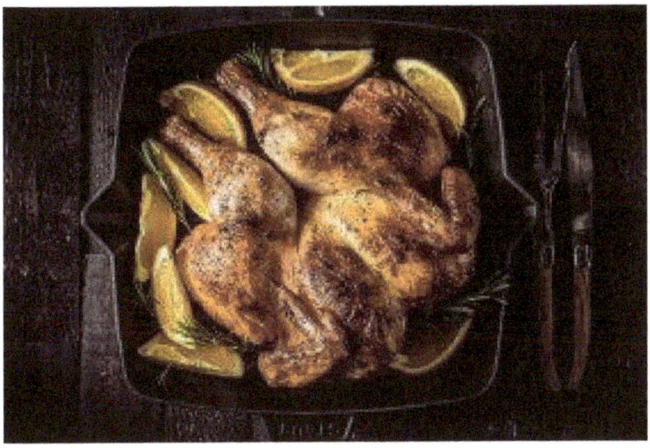

PREP TIME

15 MINS

COOK TIME

45 MINS

SERVES

4-6

HARDWOOD

MAPLE

INGREDIENTS

1 (3-4 LBS) CHICKEN, BACKBONE REMOVED

1/4 CUP OLIVE OIL

2 ORANGES, DIVIDED

ZEST OF 1 ORANGE

2 TSP DIJON MUSTARD

3 TBSP CHOPPED ROSEMARY LEAVES

2 TSP KOSHER SALT

PREPARATION

Rinse the chicken and pat dry with paper towels.

For the Marinade: In a medium bowl, combine the olive oil, juice from the oranges (about 1/4 cup of freshly squeezed juice), the orange zest, dijon mustard, rosemary leaves and salt. Whisk to combine.

Place the chicken in a shallow baking dish large enough to be fully opened in one piece.

Pour the marinade over the chicken ensuring it is covered with the marinade. Cover with plastic wrap and refrigerate for a minimum of 2 hours or up to overnight, turning once during the process.

When ready to cook, set temperature to 350°F and preheat, lid closed for 15 minutes.

Remove the chicken from the marinade and place on the grill, skin side down. Cook for 25-30 minutes until the skin is well-browned, then flip.

Continue to grill chicken until the internal temperature of the breast reaches 165°F and the thigh reaches 175°F, about 5-15 minutes longer.

Let rest 10 minutes before carving. Enjoy!

LOADED GRILLED CHICKEN TACOS

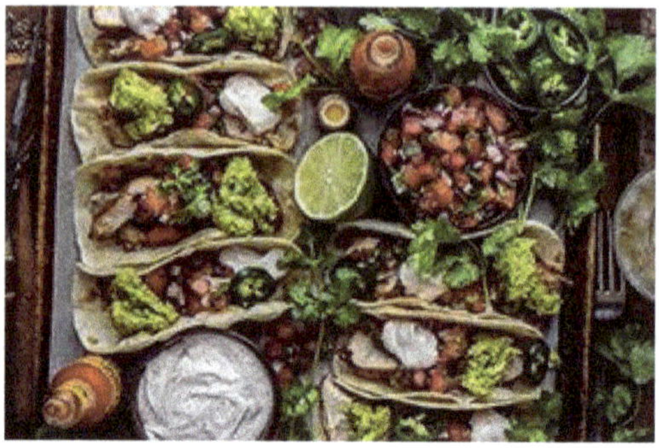

PREP TIME

4.5 HRS

COOK TIME

30 MINS

SERVES

4-6

HARDWOOD

CHERRY

INGREDIENTS

GRILLED CHICKEN

2 LBS BONELESS-SKINLESS CHICKEN BREASTS

2 TBSP OLIVE OIL

2 TSP CHILI POWDER

1 TSP SMOKED PAPRIKA

1/2 TSP GROUND CUMIN

1/4 TSP GROUND CAYENNE

1 1/2 TSP KOSHER SALT KOSHER SALT

1 TSP FRESH CRACKED BLACK PEPPER

PICO DE GALLO

1 1/2 LBS RIPE PLUM TOMATOES, DICED

1 MEDIUM RED ONION, DICED

1/2 CUP FRESH CILANTRO LEAVES, CHOPPED

JUICE OF 1 LIME

KOSHER SALT, TO TASTE

GUACAMOLE

2 RIPE AVOCADOS

1 TBSP FRESH SQUEEZED LIME JUICE

1/4 CUP FINELY DICED RED ONION

2 TBSP FINELY CHOPPED CILANTRO LEAVES

KOSHER SALT, TO TASTE

SPIKED SOUR CREAM

1/2 CUP SOUR CREAM

1 TSP CHILI POWDER

1 TBSP FRESH SQUEEZED LIME JUICE

PINCH OF KOSHER SALT

TOPPINGS

10-12 FLOUR TORTILLAS

1 LIME, CUT INTO WEDGES

1-2 JALAPENOS, SLICED

HANDFUL OF FRESH CILANTRO

HOT SAUCE

PREPARATION

For the Marinade: Combine the chicken breasts, olive oil, spices, zest, salt, and pepper in freezer bag and give everything a good mix. Chill in the fridge for at least 4 hours (overnight is best).

When ready to cook, set temperature to High and preheat, lid closed for 15 minutes.

Place the chicken breasts on the hot grill and cook, lid closed, for 25 to 30 minutes, until crispy, golden, and the chicken reaches an internal temperature of 165°F.

Rest the grilled chicken for 5 minutes before slicing into thin strips.

While the chicken is on the grill, prepare the pico, guacamole, and spiked sour cream.

For the Pico: Combine all the pico ingredients in a small bowl and mix well. Set aside.

For the Guacamole: Peel and carefully remove the pit from the avocados. Smash the avocado in a bowl until smooth, leaving a few chunks for texture, then add the remaining guacamole ingredients and give everything a good mix.

For the Spiked Sour Cream: Combine all the spiked sour cream ingredients in a small bowl and mix well.

Divide the sliced grilled chicken on warm tortillas, then hit each with fresh pico, guacamole, and a dollop of spiked-sour cream.

Top each taco with sliced jalapeño and fresh cilantro, and serve with lime wedges and hot sauce. Enjoy!

GRILLED THAI CHICKEN BURGERS WITH PAPAYA SLAW

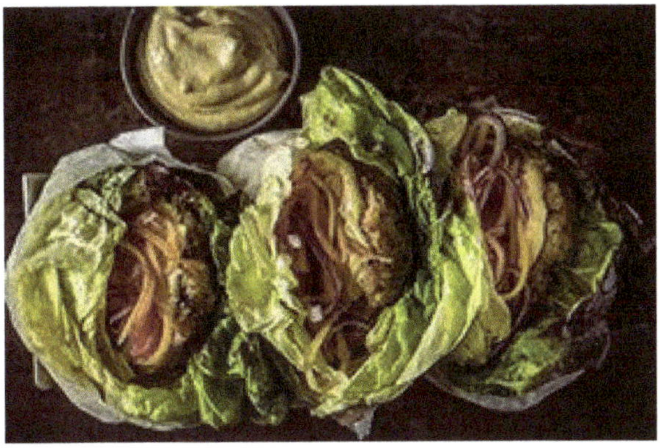

PREP TIME

40 MINS

COOK TIME

10 MINS

SERVES

6-8

HARDWOOD

HICKORY

INGREDIENTS

PAPAYA SLAW

6 OZ SHREDDED GREEN PAPAYA (FROM 1 MEDIUM PAPAYA)

1/2 RED ONION, THINLY SLICED

2 TSP GRATED LIME ZEST

3 TBSP PLUS 2 TSP FRESH LIME JUICE

1 TBSP FISH SAUCE

1 TBSP BROWN SUGAR

CHICKEN BURGER

1 LB GROUND CHICKEN THIGH MEAT

1/2 CUP PANKO OR GLUTEN FREE BREAD CRUMBS

1/4 CUP COCONUT CREAM (THICK MILK SOLIDS FROM 1 CAN CHILLED COCONUT MILK)

1/2 CUP CHOPPED FRESH CILANTRO

2 GARLIC CLOVES, MINCED

2 TSP KOSHER SALT

1 TSP GROUND CUMIN

1 TSP FRESHLY GROUND BLACK PEPPER

1/2 TSP GROUND GINGER

1/2 CUP MAYONNAISE

1 1/2 TSP CURRY POWDER

1 TBSP VEGETABLE OIL

8 LARGE LEAVES BUTTER LETTUCE OR 4 HAMBURGER BUNS

PREPARATION

For the Papaya Slaw: In a medium bowl, combine the papaya, onion, 3 Tbsp of the lime juice, fish sauce and the brown sugar. Cover and refrigerate until ready to use, up to 3 hours.

In a large bowl, stir together the ground chicken, breadcrumbs, coconut cream, cilantro, garlic, ginger, salt, pepper, cumin, lime zest, and remaining 2 tsp lime juice until thoroughly combined. Refrigerate for 20 minutes. If the mixture seems too wet or dry adjust with breadcrumbs or coconut milk until it stays together.

Meanwhile, in a small bowl, stir together the mayonnaise and curry powder. Set aside.

When ready to cook, set temperature to High and preheat, lid closed for 15 minutes.

Using your hands, form the chicken mixture into four equal patties.

Brush each burger with the vegetable oil on both sides. Cook for 4-5 minutes per side, or until the burgers reach 165°F internally. Remove from the grill and allow to rest for a few minutes before serving.

Place each burger on a leaf of lettuce then top with curry mayonnaise and pickled papaya slaw. Top with a second lettuce leaf and serve.

Alternatively, use regular hamburger buns and pile high with the burgers, curry mayonnaise and papaya slaw. Enjoy!

BAKED BUFFALO CHICKEN DIP

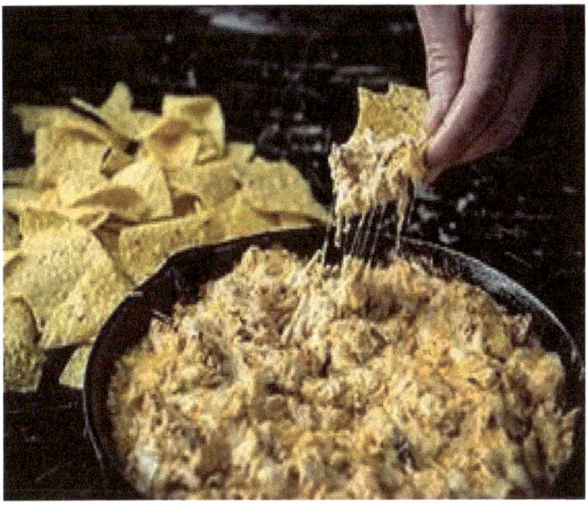

PREP TIME

10 MINS

COOK TIME

30 MINS

SERVES

6-8

HARDWOOD

MESQUITEINGREDIENTS

INGREDIENTS

1 (8 OZ) PACKAGE CREAM CHEESE, SOFTENED
1/2 CUP SOUR CREAM
1/2 CUP MAYONNAISE
2 TBSP DRY RANCH SEASONING
1 TSP KOSHER SALT
1/2 CUP FRANKS RED HOT SAUCE
2 CUPS CHICKEN, COOKED AND SHREDDED
1 CUP CHEDDAR CHEESE, SHREDDED
1 CUP MOZZARELLA CHEESE, SHREDDED
BLUE CHEESE, TO TASTE
CRUMBLED BACON, TO TASTE

PREPARATION

When ready to cook start the Traeger grill on Smoke with the lid open until fire is established (4-5 minutes). Set the temperature to 350 degrees F and preheat, lid closed for 10-15 minutes.

In the bowl of a stand mixer, combine cream cheese, sour cream, mayonnaise, ranch, salt, and hot sauce and mix with the paddle attachment until combined.

Fold together the cheddar and mozzarella cheese and shredded chicken. Transfer to an oven proof dish and top with blue cheese and crumbled bacon.

Place directly on the grill grate and cook for 20-30 minutes until the top is golden brown and dip is bubbling.

Serve with chips, crackers, crostini, or sliced vegetables. Enjoy!

TOMATILLO BRAISED CHICKEN

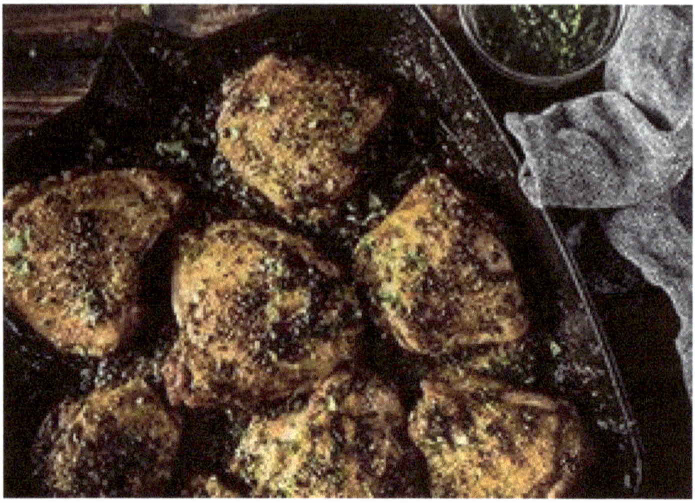

PREP TIME

20 MINS

COOK TIME

2 HRS

SERVES

4-6

HARDWOOD

HICKORY

INGREDIENTS

TOMATILLO SALSA

1 LB TOMATILLOS, HUSKS REMOVED AND RINSED

1 WHITE ONION, QUARTERED THROUGH THE ROOT END AND SKIN REMOVED

3 JALAPEÑOS, HALVED LENGTHWISE, SEEDED IF PREFERRED

2 TBSP OLIVE OIL

KOSHER SALT

3 TBSP LIME JUICE

2 TBSP CHOPPED CILANTRO

BRAISED CHICKEN

8 BONE-IN, SKIN-ON CHICKEN THIGHS

6 BONE-IN, SKIN-ON CHICKEN BREASTS

KOSHER SALT

FRESHLY GROUND PEPPER

1/2 CUP CHICKEN STOCK

2 CUPS TOMATILLO SALSA

PREPARATION

When ready to cook, set the temperature to 350°F and preheat, lid closed for 15 minutes.

Place the tomatillos, onion, and jalapeños in a large bowl and add the olive oil and 1/2 tsp salt. Toss to coat evenly, then place in a grilling basket or a baking sheet.

Grill, turning the vegetables occasionally, until they begin to char and soften, about 5 to 10 minutes. Remove the vegetables from the grill as they are ready.

Transfer to the same bowl to catch their juices and allow them to cool to room temperature.

Place the cooled vegetables along with their juices in a blender and add the lime juice, cilantro, and another pinch of salt. Pulse until the mixture reaches the texture of a salsa. Taste, adding more salt or lime juice as desired.

Rinse the chicken and pat dry with paper towels. Sprinkle with salt and pepper on both sides.

Place the chicken skin side down on the grill grate and cook until the skin is golden brown and very crispy, 10-15 minutes. Turn, cooking the other side for 5 minutes, then transfer the chicken to a plate.

Place the grilled chicken legs in a dutch oven or cast iron and add chicken stock and salsa verde. Cover the pan and place directly on the grill grate.

Cook for 1 1/2 to 2 hours until the chicken is fork tender. Enjoy!

GRILLED STICKY GINGER CHICKEN THIGHS

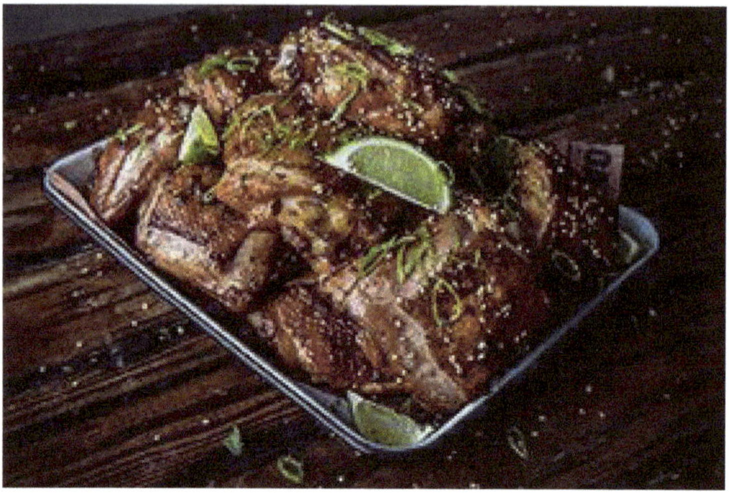

PREP TIME

10 MINS

COOK TIME

25 MINS

SERVES

4-6

HARDWOOD

PECAN

INGREDIENTS

MARINADE

1/2 CUP GRATED ONION

1/2 CUP PEANUT OIL

1/3 CUP RICE VINEGAR

2 TBSP WATER

2 TBSP GRATED FRESH GINGER

2 TBSP KETCHUP

4 TSP SOY SAUCE

2 TSP SUGAR

2 TSP LEMON JUICE

1/2 TSP MINCED GARLIC

CHICKEN THIGHS

4-6 CHICKEN THIGHS

3 GREEN ONION STALKS

2 LIMES

SESAME SEEDS, TO GARNISH

PREPARATION

Combine all sauce ingredients in a large bowl and set aside.

Place chicken thighs into a zip lock bag and add approximately 3/4 of the dressing to cover. Place in the refrigerator to marinate for at least 1 hour.

When ready to cook, set temperature to High and preheat, lid closed for 15 minutes.

Place marinated chicken thighs on the grill grate, skin side down. Cook for 10 minutes, flip and cook another 10 minutes.

Cut limes and green onions and place on chicken. Cook for an additional 5 minutes. Enjoy!

BBQ GAME DAY CHICKEN WINGS AND THIGHS

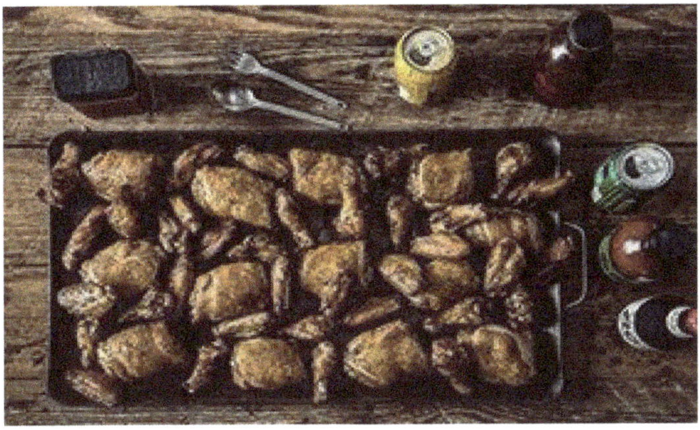

PREP TIME

3 HRS

COOK TIME

50 MINS

SERVES

6-8

HARDWOOD

CHERRY

INGREDIENTS

8-10 CHICKEN THIGHS

20-30 CHICKEN WINGS

1/2 CUP OLIVE OIL

1/2 CUP TRAEGER CHICKEN RUB

PREPARATION

When ready to cook, set the Traeger to 375°F and preheat, lid closed for 15 minutes.

Place thighs and wings in a large bowl. Add the olive oil and Traeger Chicken rub and mix well. Cover bowl and refrigerate for 3 to 8 hours.

Place chicken directly on the grill grate and cook for 45 minutes. Check the internal temperature of the chicken, it is considered done at 165°F however, a finished temperature of 175 to 180°F results in a better texture in dark meat.

Once the finished temperature is reached, remove chicken from the grill and let rest for 5 to 10 minutes before serving. Enjoy!

BAKED GARLIC PARMESAN WINGS

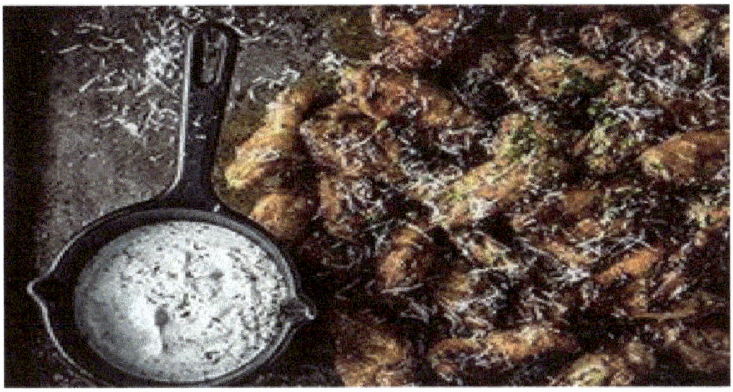

PREP TIME

10 MINS

COOK TIME

30 MINS

SERVES

4-6

HARDWOOD

CHERRY

INGREDIENTS

CHICKEN WINGS

5 LBS CHICKEN WINGS

1/2 CUP TRAEGER CHICKEN RUB

SAUCE

1 CUP BUTTER

10 CLOVES GARLIC, FINELY DICED

2 TBSP TRAEGER CHICKEN RUB

GARNISH

1 CUP PARMESAN CHEESE, SHREDDED

3 TBSP PARSLEY, CHOPPED

PREPARATION

When ready to cook, set temperature to High and preheat, lid closed for 15 minutes.

In a large bowl, toss the wings with the Traeger Chicken rub.

Place wings directly on the grill grate and cook for 10 minutes. Flip wings and cook for an additional 10 minutes. Check the internal temperature of the wings, finished desired temperature is 165-180 degrees F.

To make the Garlic Sauce: While the chicken is cooking, combine butter, garlic and remaining rub in a medium sized saucepan and cook over medium heat on a stove top. Cook sauce for 8-10 minutes, stirring occasionally.

When wings are finished cooking, remove from grill and place in a large bowl. Toss wings with the garlic sauce, parmesan cheese and parsley. Enjoy!

ROASTED HABANERO WINGS

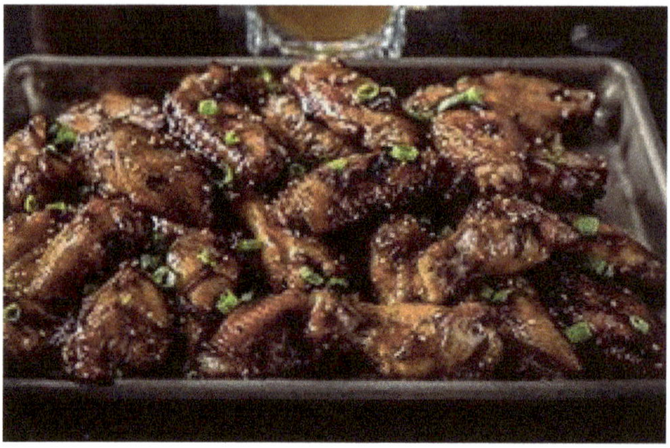

PREP TIME

6 HRS

COOK TIME

60 MINS

SERVES

4-6

HARDWOOD

HICKORY

INGREDIENTS

4 LBS CHICKEN WINGS

1 WHITE ONION, PEELED AND CHOPPED

2/3 CUP SLICED GREEN ONIONS, WHITE AND LIGHT GREEN PARTS ONLY, PLUS 2 TBSP FOR GARNISH

2 CLOVES GARLIC, PEELED AND MINCED

1/4 CUP VEGETABLE OIL

2 TBSP LOW-SODIUM SOY SAUCE OR TAMARI

2 TBSP HABANERO OR OTHER HOT PEPPER SAUCE

1-1/2 TSP SALT

1-1/2 TSP GROUND ALLSPICE

1 TSP GROUND BLACK PEPPER

1/2 TSP DRIED THYME

1/2 TSP GROUND CINNAMON

1 HABANERO PEPPER, SEEDS REMOVED

PREPARATION

Cut off the tips of the wings and discard or save for making stock. Cut the wings into drumette and flat sections.

To make the Marinade: Combine the onion, green onions and scallions in a food processor and puree until it is the texture of a thick paste. Add the oil, soy sauce, hot pepper sauce, the salt and all of the spices, and half or all of the habanero pepper, depending on how much heat you prefer. Process until all ingredients are combined. Reserve some of the marinade for basting and set aside.

Arrange the wings in a shallow baking dish and pour the marinade over the wings, tossing with tongs to ensure wings are evenly coated in sauce. Cover and refrigerate wings. Allow them to marinate for at least 6 hours or up to overnight, turning the wings at least twice.

When ready to cook, set the Traeger to 350°F and preheat, lid closed for 15 minutes.

Remove the wings from the marinade and discard what is left of the marinade.

Place the wings directly on the grill grate and cook for 30 minutes, baste the wings with the reserved marinade and flip.

Close the lid and continue cooking for another 20 minutes, or until the wings are browned and crispy and have reached an internal temperature of at least 165°F.

Garnish wings with the remaining green onions and serve immediately. Enjoy!

SMOKED CHICKEN TIKKA DRUMSTICKS

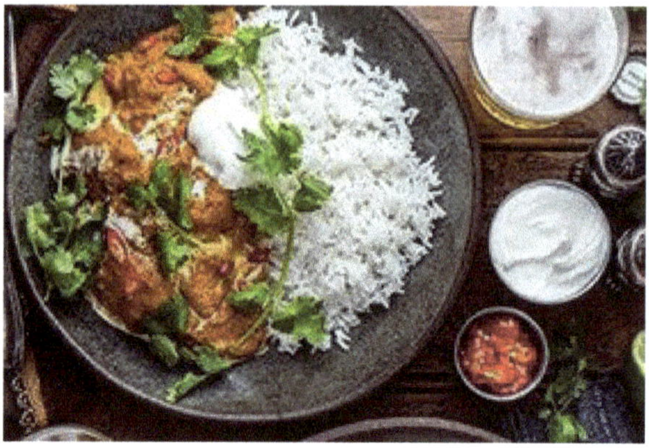

PREP TIME

10 MINS

COOK TIME

45 MINS

SERVES

6-8

HARDWOOD

MESQUITE

INGREDIENTS

CHICKEN TIKKA DRUMSTICKS

1 TBSP SMOKED PAPRIKA

1 TBSP GARAM MASALA

1 TBSP GROUND CUMIN

1 TBSP GROUND CORIANDER

1 TSP TURMERIC

1 TSP GROUND CAYENNE

1/2 MEDIUM SPANISH ONION, DICED

1 THUMB-SIZED PIECE OF GINGER, PEELED AND ROUGHLY CHOPPED

6 CLOVES GARLIC, CHOPPED

1/2 CUP GREEK YOGURT

JUICE OF 1/2 A LEMON

1/4 CUP OLIVE OIL

12 CHICKEN DRUMSTICKS

CURRY LIME YOGURT

1-1/2 CUPS GREEK YOGURT

1 TBSP CURRY POWDER

1 TBSP FRESH SQUEEZED LIME JUICE

PINCH OF SEA SALT

GARNISHES

FRESH CILANTRO

1/2 SMALL RED ONION, THINLY SLICED

1 LIME, CUT INTO WEDGES

1-2 SLICED GREEN OR RED CHILIES

PREPARATION

For the Marinade: In the base of a food processor, combine the spices, ginger, garlic, onion, yogurt, lemon juice, oil, and salt, and pulse until smooth.

Place the chicken in a large bowl, pour over the marinade, then massage chicken until every nook and cranny of the chicken is coated. Cover with plastic wrap and chill in the fridge overnight (at least 12 hours).

When ready to cook, set the temperature to High and preheat, lid closed for 15 minutes.

Place the chicken directly on the grill grates and cook for 45-50 minutes, until crispy and wood-fire grilled to perfection (or until it reaches an internal temperature of 165°F).

For the Curry Lime Yogurt: While the chicken is grilling, combine all of the yogurt ingredients in a small bowl and mix well. Chill in the fridge until ready to serve.

Garnish with fresh cilantro and sliced red onion and serve with curry lime yoghurt, fresh lime wedges, and if you like it extra spicy, sliced chilies. Enjoy!

SMOKED WILD TURKEY BREAST

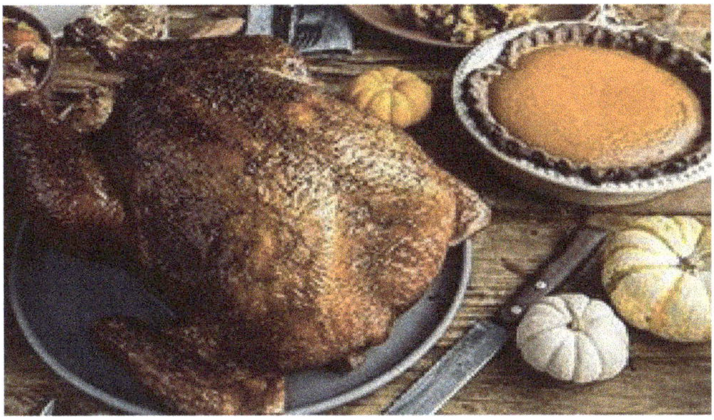

PREP TIME

12 HOURS

COOK TIME

8 HRS

SERVES

4-6

HARDWOOD

APPLE

INGREDIENTS

BRINE

2 LBS TURKEY BREAST AND DEBONED THIGH, TIED WITH SKIN ON

1 CUP BROWN SUGAR

1/4 CUP SALT

2 TBSP CRACKED PEPPER

4 CUPS COLD WATER

BBQ RUB

2 TBSP GARLIC POWDER

2 TBSP ONIONS, DRIED

2 TBSP BLACK PEPPER

2 TBSP BROWN SUGAR

1 TBSP CAYENNE PEPPER

2 TBSP CHILI POWDER

1/4 CUP PAPRIKA

1 TBSP SALT

2 TBSP SUGAR

2 TBSP CUMIN, GROUND

PREPARATION

For the Brine: In a large glass bowl combine brown sugar, salt, pepper and water. Add turkey and weigh down to completely submerge if necessary. Transfer to the refrigerator and brine for 12-24 hours.

Remove turkey from the brine and discard the brine.

When ready to cook, set the temperature 180°F and preheat lid closed for 15 minutes.

Combine ingredients for the BBQ Rub. Season turkey with rub and place directly on the grill grate skin side up.

Smoke for 5-8 hours or until the internal temperature reaches 160°F degrees when an instant read thermometer is inserted into the center.

Remove from the smoker and let rest for 10 minutes. Turkey will continue to cook once taken off grill to reach a final temperature of 165°F in the breast.

Slice and serve with your favorite sides. Enjoy!

LEMON ROSEMARY BEER CAN CHICKEN

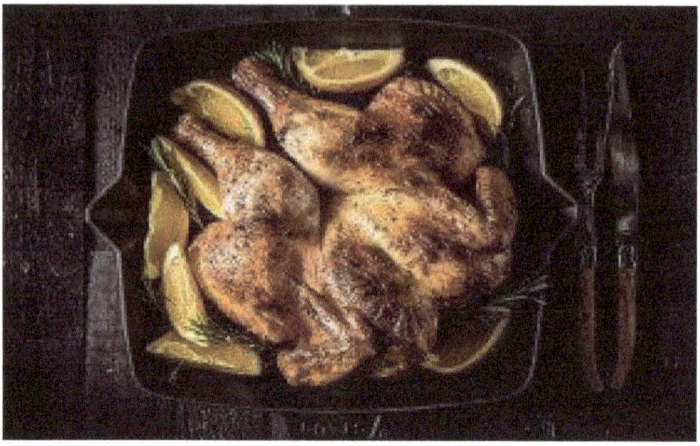

PREP TIME

5 MINS

COOK TIME

60 MINS

SERVES

4-6

HARDWOOD

OAK

INGREDIENTS

1 (3-3.5 LBS) WHOLE CHICKEN

1 LEMON

1 TSP KOSHER SALT

1 TSP GROUND PEPPER

1 TSP FRESH ROSEMARY, CHOPPED FINE

1 (12 OZ) CAN BEER

PREPARATION

When ready to cook, set temperature to High and preheat, lid closed for 15 minutes.

Coat the chicken inside and out with the juice from one lemon. In a small bowl, combine the salt, pepper and rosemary and sprinkle on the inside and out of chicken.

Empty half of the beer from the can and place the can on a solid surface. Place the chicken atop the beer can tucking the legs in the front.

Carefully place the chicken directly on the grill grate using the legs to support if needed. Alternatively, place the chicken atop the beer can on a sheet tray for a more stable surface, then place the sheet tray directly on the grill grate.

Cook the chicken until an instant read thermometer reads 165°F when inserted in the thickest part of the breast, about 60 minutes.

Let the chicken rest 10 minutes before carving.

Serve with Chardonnay or any of your favorite medium body red or white wines. Enjoy!

TURKEY

GRILLED WILD TURKEY ORANGE CASHEW SALAD

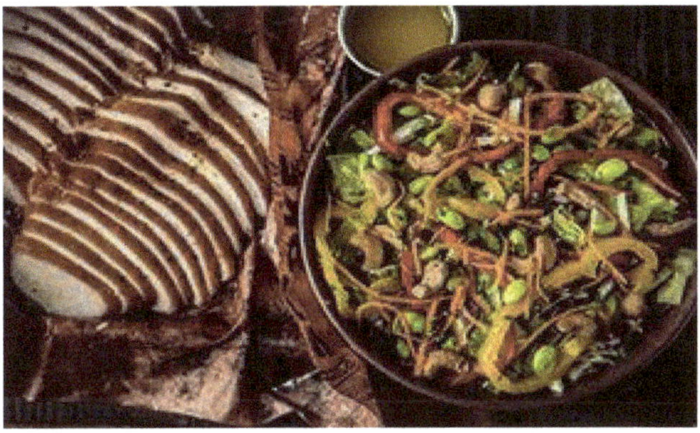

PREP TIME

6 HRS

COOK TIME

45 MINS

SERVES

4-6

HARDWOOD

PECAN

INGREDIENTS

TURKEY BREAST

2 WILD TURKEY BREAST HALVES, WITHOUT SKIN

1/4 CUP TERIYAKI SAUCE

1 TSP FRESH GINGER

1 (12 OZ) CAN BLOOD ORANGE KILL CLIFF OR SIMILAR CITRUS SODA

2 TBSP TRAEGER CHICKEN RUB

CASHEW SALAD

4 CUPS ROMAINE LETTUCE, CHOPPED

1/2 HEAD RED OR WHITE CABBAGE, CHOPPED

1/2 CUP SHREDDED CARROTS

1/2 CUP EDAMAME, SHELLED

1 SMOKED YELLOW BELL PEPPER, SLICED INTO CIRCLES

1 SMOKED RED BELL PEPPER, SLICED INTO CIRCLES

3 CHIVE TIPS, CHOPPED

1/2 CUP SMOKED CASHEWS

BLOOD ORANGE VINAIGRETTE

1 TSP ORANGE ZEST

JUICE FROM 1/2 LARGE ORANGE

1 TSP FINELY GRATED FRESH GINGER

2 TBSP SEASONED RICE VINEGAR

1 TSP HONEY

SEA SALT, TO TASTE

1/4 CUP LIGHT VEGETABLE OIL

PREPARATION

For the Marinade: Combine teriyaki sauce, Kill Cliff soda and fresh ginger. Pour marinade over turkey breasts in a Ziplock bag or dish and seal. Marinate in the refrigerator for 6 to 24 hours, turning occasionally.

When ready to cook, set temperature to to 375°F and preheat, lid closed for 15 minutes.

Remove turkey from the refrigerator, drain the marinade and pat turkey dry with paper towels.

Place turkey into a shallow oven proof dish and season with Traeger Chicken Rub.

Place dish in the Traeger and cook for 30-45 minutes or until the breast reaches an internal temperature of 160°F.

Remove the breast from the grill and wrap in Traeger Butcher Paper. Let turkey rest for 10 minutes. While turkey is resting, prepare salad.

Assemble salad ingredients in a bowl and toss to mix. Combine all ingredients in list for vinaigrette.

After resting for 10 minutes, slice turkey and serve with cashew salad and blood orange vinaigrette. Enjoy!

ULTIMATE TRAEGER THANKSGIVING SANDWICH

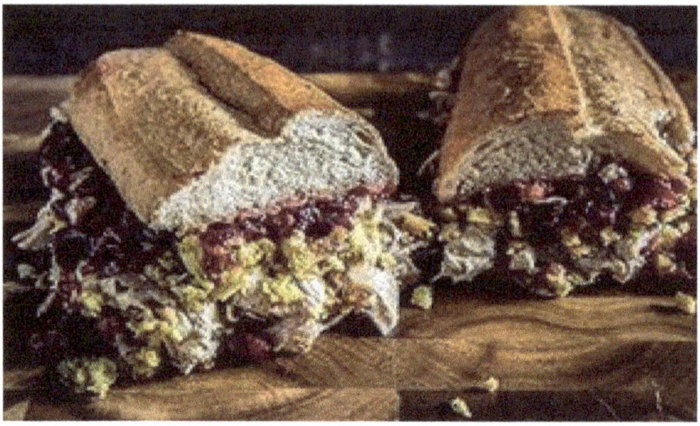

PREP TIME

10 MINS

COOK TIME

0 MINS

SERVES

2-4

HARDWOOD

TURKEY BLEND

INGREDIENTS

1 FRENCH BREAD LOAF

MAYONNAISE

DIJON MUSTARD

LEFTOVER TURKEY GRAVY

LEFTOVER SMOKED TURKEY

SHREDDED WHITE CHEDDAR CHEESE

LEFTOVER STUFFING

CRANBERRY SAUCE

PREPARATION

Slice french bread loaf in half and toast on the grill if desired. Spread mayonnaise and Dijon mustard on both halves of the bread.

Mix to combine leftover smoked turkey and gravy. Layer on top of one bread half.

Layer remaining ingredients in this order: shredded white cheddar cheese, stuffing and cranberry sauce.

Top sandwich with other bread half. Slice in half to serve. Enjoy!

BAKED CORNBREAD TURKEY TAMALE PIE

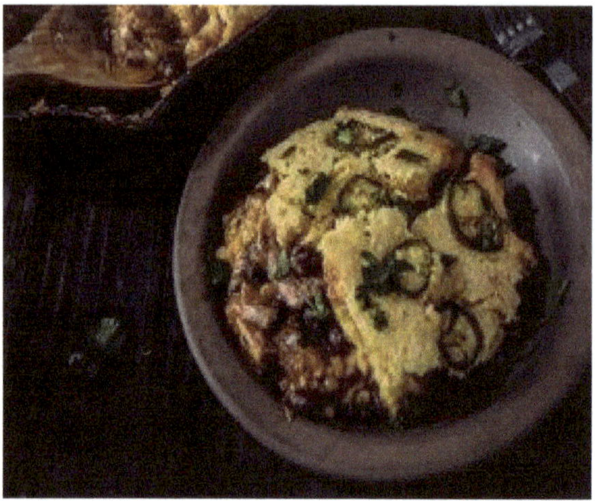

PREP TIME

10 MINS

COOK TIME

50 MINS

SERVES

6-8

HARDWOOD

TURKEY BLEND

INGREDIENTS

FILLING

2 CUPS SHREDDED TURKEY

2 COBS OF CORN

1 (15 OZ) CAN BLACK BEANS, RINSED AND DRAINED

1 YELLOW BELL PEPPER

1 ORANGE BELL PEPPER

2 JALAPEÑOS

2 TBSP CILANTRO

1 BUNCH GREEN ONIONS

1/2 TSP CUMIN

1/2 TSP PAPRIKA

1 (7 OZ) CAN CHIPOTLE SAUCE

1 (15 OZ) CAN ENCHILADA SAUCE

1/2 CUP SHREDDED CHEDDAR CHEESE

CORNBREAD TOPPING

1 CUP ALL-PURPOSE FLOUR

1 CUP YELLOW OR WHITE CORNMEAL

1 TBSP SUGAR

2 TSP BAKING POWDER

1/2 TSP SALT

3 TBSP BUTTER

1 CUP BUTTERMILK

1 LARGE EGG, LIGHTLY BEATEN

PREPARATION

For the filling: Mix to combine filling ingredients. Place in the bottom of a butter greased 10-inch pan.

For the cornbread topping: In a mixing bowl, combine the flour, cornmeal, sugar, baking powder, and salt. Melt the butter in a small saucepan. Remove butter from the heat and stir in the milk and egg. Make sure the mixture isn't too hot or the egg will curdle.

Add the milk-egg mixture to the dry ingredients and stir to combine. Do not over mix.

To assemble Tamale Pie: Fill the bottom of a butter greased 10-inch pan with the shredded turkey filling. Top with the cornbread topping and smooth to the edges of pan.

When ready to cook, set the temperature to 375°F and preheat, lid closed for 15 minutes.

Place directly on the grill grate and cook for 45-50 minutes or until the cornbread is lightly browned and cooked through. Enjoy!

BAKED THANKSGIVING SHEPHERD'S PIE

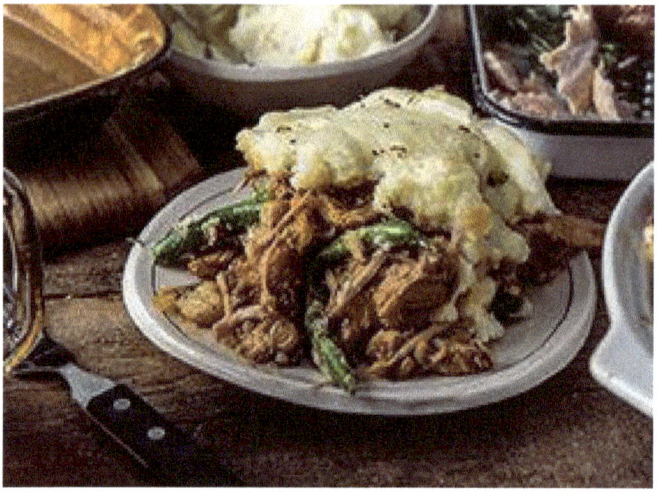

PREP TIME

10 MINS

COOK TIME

60 MINS

SERVES

6-8

HARDWOOD

APPLE

INGREDIENTS

1LB GROUND BEEF

2 CUPS LEFTOVER MASHED POTATOES

1 CUP LEFTOVER GREEN BEANS

1 CUP LEFTOVER STUFFING

1 CUP LEFTOVER GRAVY

1 1/2 LB LEFTOVER TURKEY

2 TBSP CANOLA OIL

1 CUP CHOPPED ONIONS

2 CLOVES GARLIC, MINCED

1 TSP KOSHER SALT

1/2 TSP FRESHLY GROUND BLACK PEPPER

2 TBSP ALL-PURPOSE FLOUR

2 TSP TOMATO PASTE

1 CUP CHICKEN BROTH

1 TSP WORCESTERSHIRE SAUCE

2 TSP FRESHLY CHOPPED ROSEMARY LEAVES

1 TSP FRESHLY CHOPPED THYME

PREPARATION

When ready to cook, set temperature to High and preheat, lid closed for 15 minutes.

Place canola oil in a medium sauté pan over medium-high heat. Once the oil shimmers, add the onion and sauté just until softened and lightly brown, about 3-4 minutes. Add the garlic and stir to combine.

Add the beef, salt and pepper and cook until browned and cooked through, approximately 3 minutes.

Sprinkle the onions with the flour and toss to coat, continuing to cook for another minute. Add the tomato paste, leftover gravy, chicken broth, Worcestershire, rosemary and thyme. Stir to combine.

Bring to a boil, then reduce the heat to low. Cover and simmer 10-12 minutes or until the sauce is thickened slightly.

Add the leftover turkey, green beans and stuffing to the mixture and spread evenly into an 11 x 7 inch glass baking dish.

Top with the mashed potatoes, starting around the edges to create a seal to prevent the mixture from bubbling up and smooth with a rubber spatula.

Place directly on the grill grate and bake for 25 minutes or just until the potatoes begin to brown. Remove to a cooling rack for at least 15 minutes before serving. Enjoy!

BBQ PULLED TURKEY SANDWICHES

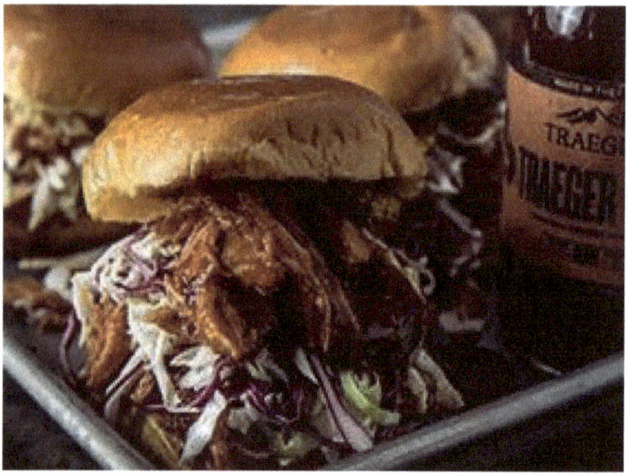

PREP TIME

15 MINS

COOK TIME

2 HRS

SERVES

6-8

HARDWOOD

MAPLE

INGREDIENTS

6 TURKEY THIGHS, SKIN-ON

1 1/2 CUPS CHICKEN OR TURKEY BROTH

TRAEGER PORK & POULTRY RUB

1 CUP TRAEGER BBQ SAUCE, OR MORE AS NEEDED

6 BUNS OR KAISER ROLLS, SPLIT AND BUTTERED

PREPARATION

Season turkey thighs on both sides with the Traeger Pork & Poultry rub.

When ready to cook, set temperature to 180°F and preheat, lid closed for 15 minutes.

Arrange the turkey thighs directly on the grill grate and smoke for 30 minutes.

Transfer the thighs to a sturdy disposable aluminum foil or roasting pan. Pour the broth around the thighs. Cover the pan with foil or a lid.

Increase temperature to 325°F and preheat, lid closed. Roast the thighs until they reach an internal temperature of 180°F.

Remove pan from the grill, but leave grill on. Let the turkey thighs cool slightly until they can be comfortably handled.

Pour off the drippings and reserve. Remove the skin and discard.

Pull the turkey meat into shreds with your fingers and return the meat to the roasting pan.

Add 1 cup or more of your favorite Traeger BBQ Sauce along with some of the drippings.

Recover the pan with foil and reheat the BBQ turkey on the Traeger for 20 to 30 minutes.

Serve with toasted buns if desired. Enjoy!

ROASTED SPATCHCOCK TURKEY

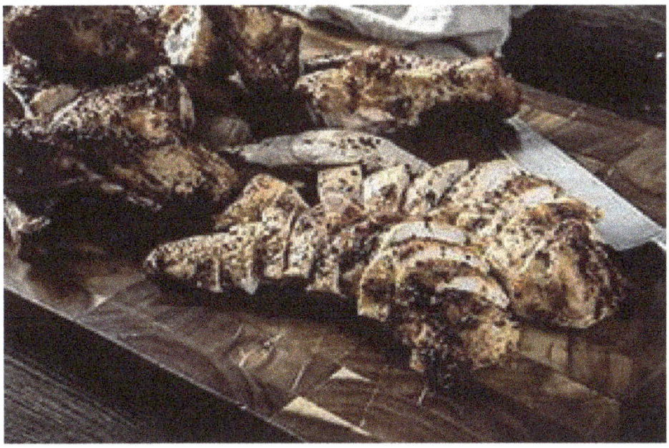

PREP TIME

30 MINS

COOK TIME

4 1/2 HRS

SERVES

8-12

HARDWOOD

TURKEY BLEND

INGREDIENTS

1 (18-20 LB) WHOLE TURKEY

4 TBSP TRAEGER TURKEY RUB

1 TBSP JACOBSEN SEA SALT
4 CLOVES GARLIC, MINCED
3 TBSP PARSLEY, CHOPPED
1 TBSP ROSEMARY, CHOPPED
2 TBSP THYME LEAVES, CHOPPED
2 SCALLIONS, CHOPPED
3 TBSP OLIVE OIL

PREPARATION

When ready to cook, set temperature to High and preheat, lid closed for 15 minutes.

On a cutting board, combine garlic, parsley, thyme, rosemary, and scallions. Chop together until the mixture forms a paste. Set aside.

To spatchcock the turkey: With a large knife or shears, cut the bird open along the backbone on both sides, through the ribs and remove the backbone.

Once the bird is open, split the breastbone to spread the bird flat; this will allow it to roast evenly.

With the bird breast side up, season the exterior with half the Traeger Turkey Rub then follow with 2/3 the herb mixture rubbing it into the bird. Drizzle with olive oil.

Flip the bird and season generously with the remaining Traeger Turkey Rub.

Place the turkey directly on the grill grate and cook for 30 minutes.

Reduce the temperature on the grill to 300°F and continue to cook for 3-4 hours or until the internal temperature reaches 160°F in the breast.

The finished internal temperature should reach 165°F, but the temperature will continue to rise after the bird is removed from the grill.

Let the bird rest 20-25 minutes before carving. Enjoy!

ROASTED CORNISH GAME STUFFED HENS

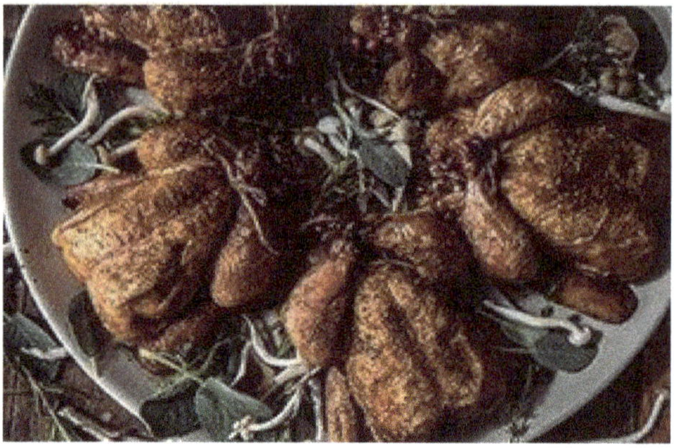

PREP TIME

10 MINS

COOK TIME

60 MINS

SERVES

4-6

HARDWOOD

APPLE

INGREDIENTS

2 TBSP BUTTER

1 PINT WILD MUSHROOMS, CLEANED

1/2 YELLOW ONION, DICED

1 STALK CELERY, DICED

1 CLOVE GARLIC, MINCED

1 CUP WILD RICE

1 1/2 CUPS CHICKEN STOCK

2 SPRIGS THYME, LEAVES REMOVED

SALT & PEPPER AS NEEDED

1/2 TBSP FRESH SAGE, MINCED

4 CORNISH GAME HENS

1/4 CUP TRAEGER FIN & FEATHER RUB

PREPARATION

Melt butter in a medium sauce pan and add wild mushrooms. Cook for 10 minutes until softened and lightly browned.

Add onion and celery and cook 5 minutes until translucent. Add garlic and cook 30 seconds more until fragrant.

Add rice and stock and bring to a simmer. Cook for about 20 minutes or until rice is tender. Add herbs and season with salt and pepper.

Stuff 1/4 to 1/2 cup of rice mixture into each bird truss the legs together. Season the exterior of the cornish game hens liberally with rub.

When ready to cook, set temperature to 375°F and preheat, lid closed for 15 minutes.

Place the birds directly on the grill grate and cook for 30 minutes or until the internal temperature registers 165°F with an instant read thermometer.

Remove from grill and let rest for a few minutes before serving. Enjoy!

SPATCHCOCKED MAPLE BRINED TURKEY

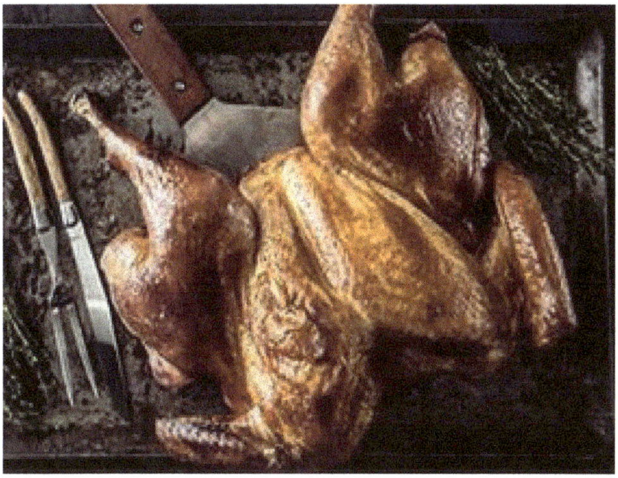

PREP TIME

8.5 HRS

COOK TIME

3 HRS

SERVES

6-8

HARDWOOD

MAPLE

INGREDIENTS

1 (12-14 LBS) TURKEY, THAWED IF FROZEN

5 QTS HOT WATER

1 1/2 CUPS KOSHER SALT

3/4 CUP BOURBON

1 CUP PURE MAPLE SYRUP

1/2 CUP BROWN SUGAR

1 ONION, PEELED AND QUARTERED THROUGH THE ROOT END

3 TO 4 STRIPS ORANGE PEEL

3 BAY LEAVES, BROKEN INTO PIECES

2 TBSP BLACK PEPPERCORNS

1 TBSP WHOLE CLOVES

3 QTS ICE

1 CUP BUTTER, MELTED

TRAEGER PORK & POULTRY RUB, AS NEEDED

SPRIGS OF FRESH SAGE AND THYME, TO GARNISH

ORANGE WEDGES, LADY APPLES, OR KUMQUATS, TO SERVE

PREPARATION

Note: Do not use a kosher turkey or a self-basting turkey for this recipe as they have already been enhanced with a salt-solution.

For the Brine: In a large stockpot or container, combine the hot water, kosher salt, bourbon, 3/4 cup of the maple syrup, brown sugar, onion, bay leaves, orange peel, peppercorns, and cloves and stir until well mixed. Add the ice.

Rinse the turkey, inside and out, under cold running water. Remove giblets and discard or save for another use. Some turkeys come with a gravy packet as well; remove it before roasting the bird.

Add the turkey to the brine and refrigerate 8 to 12 hours, or overnight. Weight with a bag of ice to keep the bird submerged.

Drain and pat dry with paper towels; discard the brine.

To spatchcock the turkey: With a large knife or shears, cut the bird open along the backbone on both sides, through the ribs and remove the backbone.

Once the bird is open, split the breastbone to spread the bird flat; this will allow it to roast evenly.

Combine the melted butter and the remaining 1/4 cup of maple syrup and divide in half. Brush half of the mixture on the bird and sprinkle with Traeger Pork & Poultry Rub or salt and black pepper.

Set aside the other half of the mixture until ready to use.

When ready to cook, set the temperature to 350°F and preheat, lid closed for 15 minutes.

Roast the turkey until the internal temperature in the thickest part of the breast reaches 165°F, about 2-3 hours.

Brush with the remaining butter-maple syrup glaze the last 30 minutes of cooking.

Let the turkey rest for 15 to 20 minutes before carving. Garnish, if desired, with fresh herbs and or kumquats. Enjoy!

ROASTED AUTUMN BRINED TURKEY BREAST

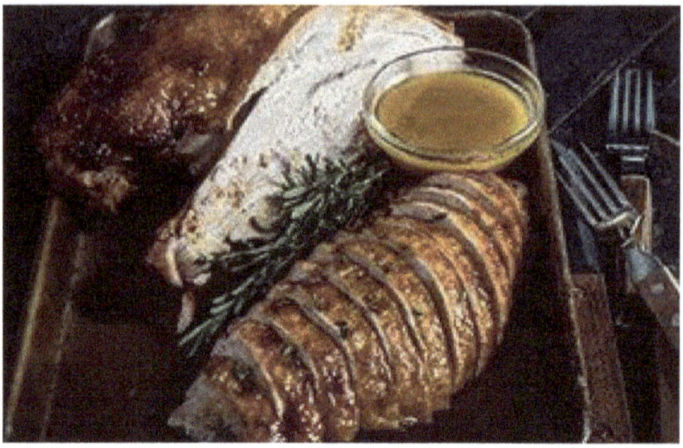

PREP TIME

8 HRS

COOK TIME

4.5 HRS

SERVES

6-8

HARDWOOD

APPLE

INGREDIENTS

6 CUPS APPLE CIDER

2 CLOVES GARLIC, SMASHED

1/3 CUP BROWN SUGAR

1 TBSP ALLSPICE

1/3 CUP KOSHER SALT

3 BAY LEAVES

4 CUPS ICE WATER

1 TURKEY BREAST

1/2 CUP PLUS TWO TBSP UNSALTED BUTTER, SOFTENED

TRAEGER PORK AND POULTRY RUB

PREPARATION

For the Brine: In a large pot, combine 4 cups of the apple cider, the garlic cloves, brown sugar, allspice, salt, and bay leaves. Simmer on stove top for 5 minutes, stirring often.

Take off stove top and add in the ice water.

Place turkey in the brine and add water as needed until the turkey is fully submerged. Cover and refrigerate overnight.

For the Cider Glaze: Boil the remaining 2 cups of apple cider in a saucepan until reduced to 1/4 cup, about 30-45 minutes. Whisk in butter and cool completely.

After turkey has brined overnight, drain turkey and rinse.

Using your fingers, take two tablespoons of the softened butter and smear it under the skin of the breast. Lightly season the turkey breast with Traeger Pork & Poultry Rub.

When ready to cook, set the temperature to 325°F and preheat, lid closed for 15 minutes.

Cook turkey until it reaches an internal temperature of 160°F, about 3-4 hrs. After the first 20 minutes of cooking, brush turkey with the cider glaze.

If the breast starts to get too dark, cover it with foil. Let stand 30 minutes before carving. Enjoy!

BAKED CHICKEN POT PIE

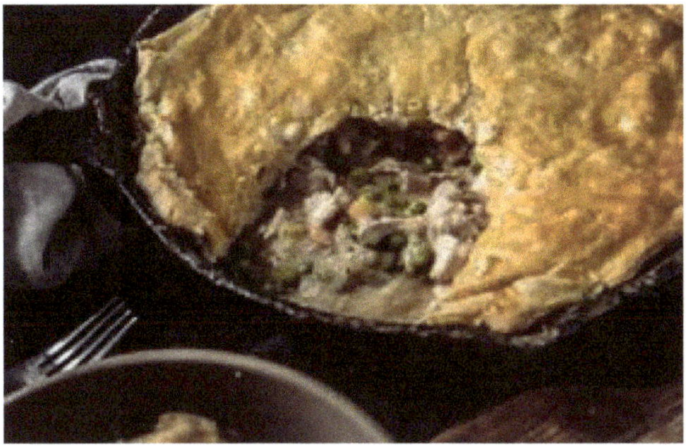

PREP TIME

20 MINS

COOK TIME

30 MINS

SERVES

4-6

HARDWOOD

HICKORY

INGREDIENTS

2 TBSP BUTTER

1 SMALL YELLOW ONION, DICED

1 STALK CELERY, DICED

2 CUPS HOMEMADE CHICKEN OR TURKEY GRAVY

1/2 CUP CREAM OR MILK

1-1/2 CUPS FROZEN PEAS AND CARROTS, THAWED

2 TSP DRY SHERRY (OPTIONAL)

1/2 TSP TRAEGER PORK & POULTRY RUB

1/4 TSP DRIED THYME LEAVES

3-4 CUPS COOKED SKINLESS CHICKEN OR TURKEY MEAT, DICED

SALT AND PEPPER, TO TASTE

FLOUR, FOR DUSTING AS NEEDED

1 SHEET FROZEN PUFF PASTRY

1 EGG, BEATEN WITH 1 TBSP WATER

PREPARATION

Melt the butter in a large saucepan over medium heat. Add the onion and celery and cook 3 to 5 minutes, or until the onion is translucent.

Stir in the gravy and cream or milk and heat gently. Add the peas and carrots, sherry, Pork and Poultry Rub, thyme leaves, and chicken and simmer for 5 to 10 minutes. Add salt and pepper to taste.

Coat cast iron skillet with cooking spray and fill with the pot pie filling.

Unroll the puff pastry sheet on a lightly floured countertop. Let thaw slightly.

Cover the top of the cast iron with the puff pastry crimping any overhang. Make several small slits in the center to let the steam escape. Brush lightly with the egg wash.

Transfer the pot pie to the grill.

Set the temperature to 400°F and preheat, lid closed for 15 minutes.

Bake the pot pie for 30 minutes, or until the puff pastry is nicely browned and the filling is bubbling. Serve immediately. Enjoy!

ROASTED HONEY BOURBON GLAZED TURKEY

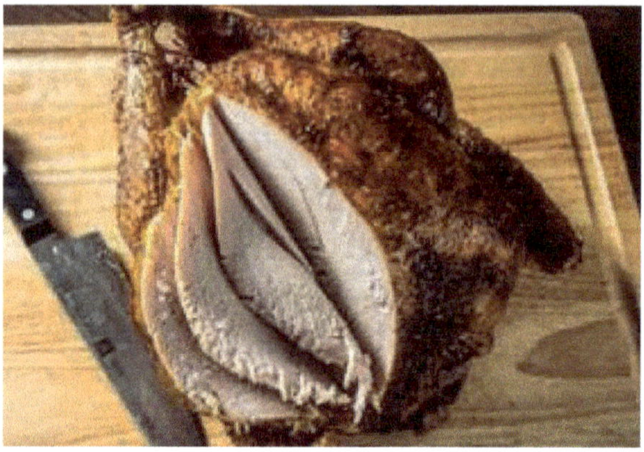

PREP TIME

30 MINS

COOK TIME

4 HRS

SERVES

8-12

HARDWOOD

MAPLE

INGREDIENTS

TURKEY

1 (16-18 LBS) TURKEY

1/4 CUP TRAEGER FIN AND FEATHER RUB

WHISKEY GLAZE

1/2 CUP BOURBON

1/2 CUP HONEY

1/4 CUP BROWN SUGAR

3 TBSP APPLE CIDER VINEGAR

1 TBSP DIJON MUSTARD

SALT AND PEPPER, TO TASTE

PREPARATION

When ready to cook, set the temperature to 375°F and preheat, lid closed for 15 minutes.

Truss the turkey legs together. Season the exterior of the bird and the cavity with Traeger Fin and Feather Rub.

Place the turkey directly on the grill grate and cook for 20-30 minutes at 375°F or until the skin begins to brown.

After 30 minutes, reduce the temperature to 325°F and continue to cook until internal temperature registers 165°F when an instant read thermometer is inserted into the thickest part of the breast, about 3-4 hours.

For the Whiskey Glaze: Combine all ingredients in a small saucepan and bring to a boil. Reduce the temperature and let simmer 15-20 minutes or until thick enough to coat the back of a spoon. Remove from heat and set aside.

During the last ten minutes of cooking, brush the glaze on the turkey while on the grill and cook until the glaze is set, about 10 minutes.

Remove from grill and let rest 10-15 minutes before carving. Enjoy!

HOMEMADE TURKEY GRAVY

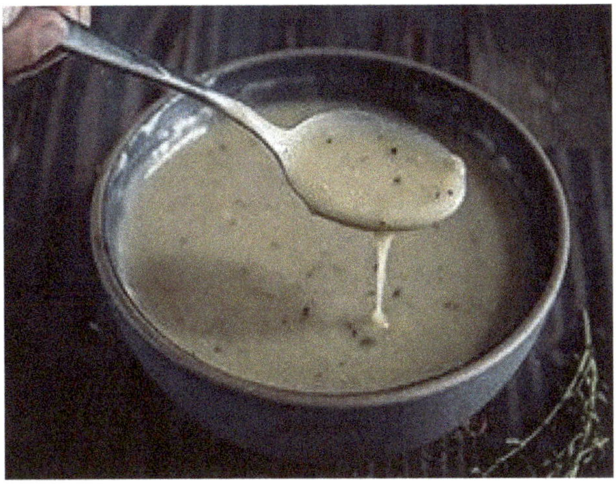

PREP TIME

20 MINS

COOK TIME

3 HRS

SERVES

8-12

HARDWOOD

APPLE

INGREDIENTS

4 CUPS HOMEMADE CHICKEN STOCK

2 LARGE ONIONS CUT INTO 8TH

4 CARROTS, ROUGH CHOP

4 CELERY STALKS

8 SPRIGS THYME

8 CLOVES GARLIC, PEELED AND SMASHED

1 TURKEY NECK

1 CUP FLOUR

1 STICK BUTTER, CUT INTO ABOUT 8 PIECES

1 TSP KOSHER SALT

1 TSP CRACKED BLACK PEPPER

PREPARATION

When ready to cook, set the temperature to 350°F and preheat with the lid closed, for 15 minutes.

In a large roasting pan, place turkey neck, onion, celery, carrot, garlic and thyme. Add 4 cups of chicken stock and sprinkle with salt and pepper.

Place the prepped turkey on the rack into the roasting pan and place in the Traeger.

Cook for 3-4 hours or until the breast reaches 160°F. Once taken off the grill, the turkey will continue to cook and will reach a finished internal temperature of 165°F.

Strain the drippings into a saucepan and simmer on low.

In a larger saucepan combine butter and flour with a whisk stirring until golden tan. This takes about 8 minutes, stirring constantly.

Next whisk the drippings into the roux and cook until it comes to a boil. Season with salt and pepper and serve hot. Enjoy!

GRILLED CHICKEN FAJITAS

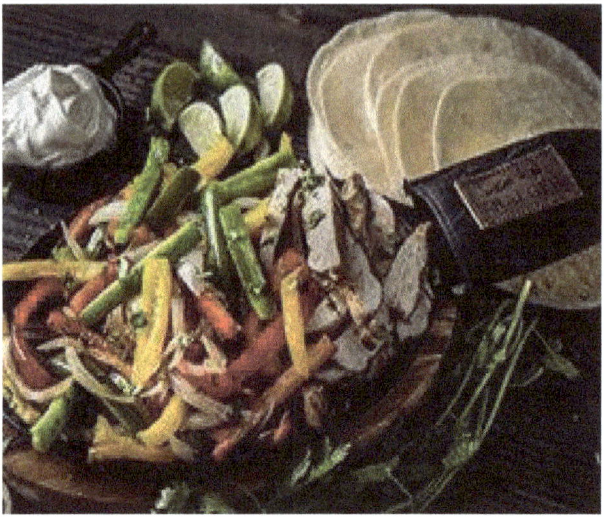

PREP TIME

60 MINS

COOK TIME

20 MINS

SERVES

2-4

HARDWOOD

MESQUITE

INGREDIENTS

CAST IRON FAJITA PLATE

2 EA BONELESS SKINLESS CHICKEN BREASTS

1/2 TBSP CUMIN

1/2 TBSP CHILI POWDER

JUICE OF 1 LIME

SALT AND PEPPER, TO TASTE

1 SMALL YELLOW ONION, SLICED

1 GREEN BELL PEPPER, SLICED

1 RED BELL PEPPER, SLICED

1 TBSP OLIVE OIL

TORTILLAS, TO SERVE

PREPARATION

Place chicken breasts in a Ziploc bag and add cumin, chili powder, lime juice and salt and pepper. Transfer to the refrigerator and marinate for 1 hour.

When ready to cook, set temperature to High and preheat, lid closed for 15 minutes.

Place fajita skillet directly on the grill grate and preheat for 30 minutes. Place olive oil in the pan and add the onions and peppers, season with salt and pepper and close the lid.

Cook 10 minutes or until lightly browned and cooked through.

Lay the chicken breast directly on the grill grate next to the skillet and cook 10-15 minutes flipping halfway through until the internal temperature reaches 165°F .

Remove chicken breast from grill and let rest before slicing.

Serve sliced chicken with peppers and onions on the fajita plate with tortillas and choice of toppings. Enjoy!

BEEF RECIPES FOR WOOD PELLET SMOKER GRILLS

TRAEGER BBQ BRISKET

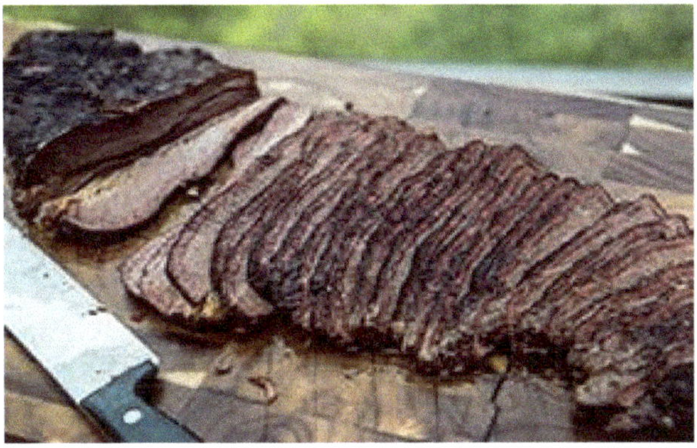

PREP TIME

12 HRS

COOK TIME

9 HRS

SERVES

8-12

HARDWOOD

HICKORY

INGREDIENTS

1 (12-14 LB) WHOLE PACKER BRISKET

TRAEGER BEEF RUB, AS NEEDED

PREPARATION

Coat meat liberally with Traeger Beef Rub. When seasoned, wrap brisket in plastic wrap. Let the wrapped meat sit 12 to 24 hours in the refrigerator.

When ready to cook, set the Traeger to 225°F and preheat, lid closed for 15 minutes.

Place meat fat side down on the grill grate and cook for 6 hours or until internal temperature reaches 160°F. Remove brisket from the grill and wrap in foil.

Place foiled brisket back on grill and cook until it reaches a finished internal temperature of 204°F this should take an additional 3-4 hours.

Remove from grill and allow to rest in the foil for at least 30 minutes. Slice. Enjoy!

GARLIC, LEMON, AND GOAT CHEESE MASHED POTATOES

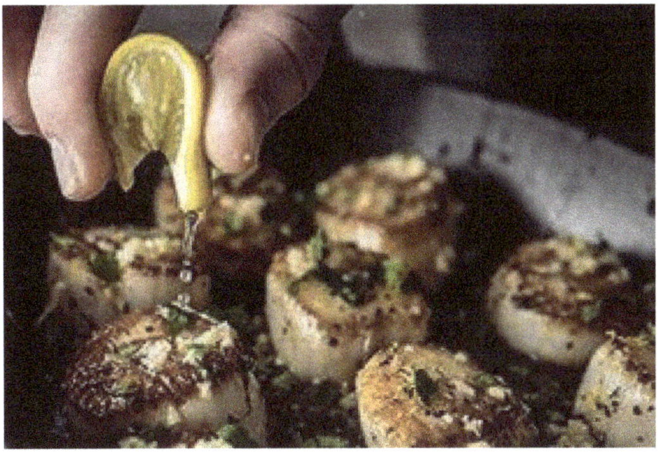

PREP TIME

10 MINS

COOK TIME

60 MINS

SERVES

8-12

HARDWOOD

HICKORY

INGREDIENTS

1 HEAD OF GARLIC

1 TSP OLIVE OIL

3 LBS YUKON GOLD POTATOES, PEELED AND ROUGHLY CHOPPED

3/4 CUP CRUMBLED GOAT CHEESE

1/4 CUP MELTED BUTTER, PLUS MORE FOR DRIZZLING

3/4 CUP HEAVY WHIPPING CREAM

SEA SALT & FRESHLY CRACKED BLACK PEPPER

2 TBS FRESH CHIVES, FINELY DICED

PREPARATION

When ready to cook, set the temperature to 350°F and preheat, lid closed, for 10 to 15 minutes.

Using a sharp knife, slice about ⅛" off the top of the garlic head (leaving the root intact), exposing the individual garlic cloves. Drizzle the olive oil on top of the exposed garlic and season with a pinch of salt and pepper. Tightly wrap the bulb in aluminum foil and roast on the Traeger for 30 - 35 minutes, until the cloves are soft. Remove the garlic cloves and mash into a paste with a fork.

Meanwhile, bring a large stockpot of salted water to a boil over medium high heat. Add the potatoes and cook for 15 - 20 minutes, or until softened and mashable. Drain and return to the pot, stirring until dry. Remove from the heat and stir in the cream, goat cheese, lemon zest, garlic mash, and ¼ cup of butter. Mash until smooth, and if you like it, whip that business up with a whisk. Season with salt and pepper to taste. Garnish with extra chives and a generous drizzle of melted butter. Enjoy!

TRAEGER PRIME RIB ROAST

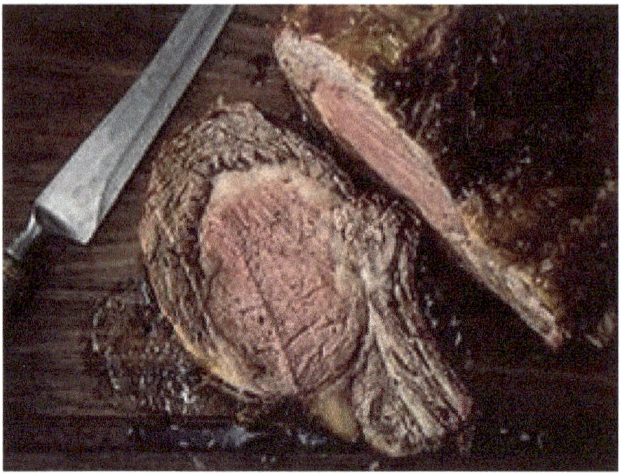

PREP TIME

24 HRS

COOK TIME

4 HRS

SERVES

8-12

HARDWOOD

CHERRY

INGREDIENTS

1 (5-7 BONES) PRIME RIB ROAST

TRAEGER PRIME RIB RUB, AS NEEDED

PREPARATION

Coat the roast evenly with the Traeger Prime Rib Rub and wrap in plastic wrap. Let sit in the refrigerator for 24 hours.

When ready to cook, set the temperature to High and preheat, lid closed for 15 minutes.

Place the prime rib fat side up, directly on the grill grate and cook for 30 minutes. Starting at a higher heat will help to develop a crispy, rendered crust.

After 30 minutes, reduce the grill temperature to 325°F.

Close lid and roast at 325°F for 3-4 hours or until cooked to desired internal temperature, 120°F for rare, 130°F for medium rare, 140°F for medium and 150°F for well done.

Remove from grill and let rest 15 minutes before carving. Enjoy!

ITALIAN BEEF SANDWICH

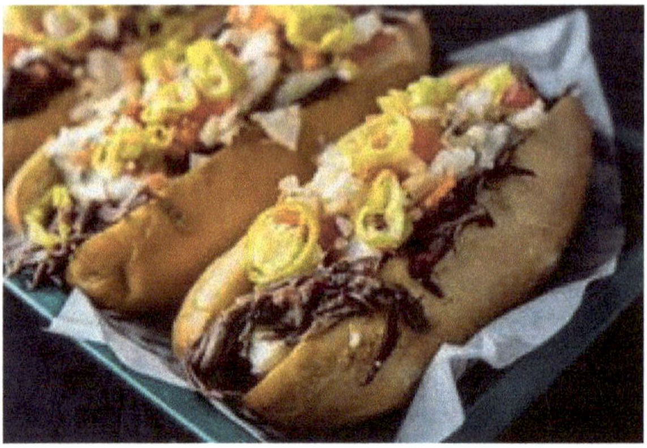

PREP TIME

20 MINS

COOK TIME

3 HRS

SERVES

6-8

HARDWOOD

ALDER

INGREDIENTS

1 QTY. (4 LB.) LEAN, BONELESS BEEF ROAST (SIRLOIN OR TOP ROUND)

SALT

PEPPER

4 CLOVES GARLIC, THINLY SLICED

TRAEGER PRIME RIB RUB

6 CUPS BEEF BROTH

8 HOAGIE-STYLE BUNS (FOR SANDWICHES)

6 SLICES SWISS CHEESE

1 CUP BOTTLED GIARDINIERA (ITALIAN PICKLED VEGETABLES; OPTIONAL), CHOPPED

PREPARATION

When ready to cook, set the temperature to 450°F and preheat, lid closed for 15 minutes.

Season the roast liberally with salt, pepper and Traeger prime rib rub. Using a paring knife, make 10-15 slits in the roast every 1″ or so. Insert a garlic clove into each slit.

Place the roast directly on the grill grate and cook for about 1 hour flipping halfway through until browned well.

Remove the roast from the grill and transfer to a deep dutch oven. Pour the beef broth over the roast.

Cover tightly with foil and place back on the grill. Reduce the grill temperature to 300°F and cook the roast for 3-4 hours or until it is fork tender.

While the roast cooks, chop the giardiniera into small pieces.

Remove the dutch oven from the grill and shred removing any large bits of fat or connective tissue. Transfer the meat back to the dutch over and stir to combine with the juices.

Increase the grill temperature to high and preheat lid closed for 10 minutes.

Place hoagie buns cut side up on a small sheet tray. Fill with the shredded roast and top with a slice of cheese. Transfer to the grill and cook for another 5-10 minutes or until the cheese is melted.

Remove from the grill and top with chopped pickled veggies. Serve with remaining cooking liquid for dipping if desired. Enjoy!

THAI BEEF SKEWERS

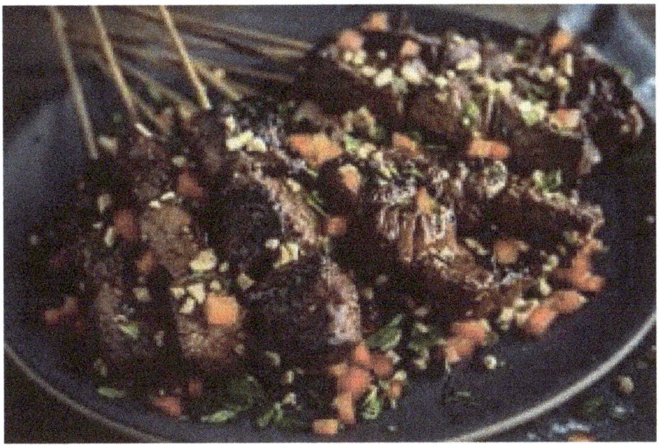

PREP TIME

15 MINS

COOK TIME

8 MIN

SERVES

4-6

HARDWOOD

CHERRY

INGREDIENTS

1/4 CUP VEGETABLE OIL

1/4 CUP SOY SAUCE

1 JUICE OF LIME

2 CLOVES GARLIC, FINELY MINCED

1 TBSP. FRESH GINGER, PEELED AND MINCED

1 TBSP. SUGAR

1 TSP. BLACK PEPPER, FRESHLY GROUND

1/2 BEEF SIRLOIN, TRIMMED AND CUT INTO 1-1/4 INCH DICE

1/2 RED BELL PEEPER, STEMMED, SEEDED, AND CUT INTO 1/4 INCH DICE

1/2 CUP DRY-ROASTED PEANUTS (SALTED OR UNSALTED), COARSELY CHOPPED

1 TRAEGER SKEWERS SET

PREPARATION

In a small bowl, whisk together the oil, soy sauce, lime juice, garlic, ginger, sugar, and black pepper. Transfer the meat to a large bowl or resealable plastic bag and pour the marinade over the meat, turning to coat each piece thoroughly. Refrigerate for 2 to 4 hours, or longer if desired.

Drain the marinade off the sirloin cubes (discard the marinade) and pat them dry with paper towels.

Thread the meat on the skewers, keeping the pieces close together to minimize exposure of the skewer to the heat. (You can also slip a folded length of aluminum foil under the exposed ends to protect them.)

When ready to cook, set the temperature to 425°F and preheat, lid closed for 15 minutes.

Arrange the skewers on the grill grate and grill for 2 to 4 minutes per side, or until the desired degree of doneness is reached. To serve, sprinkle with the diced red pepper and the chopped peanuts. Enjoy!

BBQ CHILI BURGER

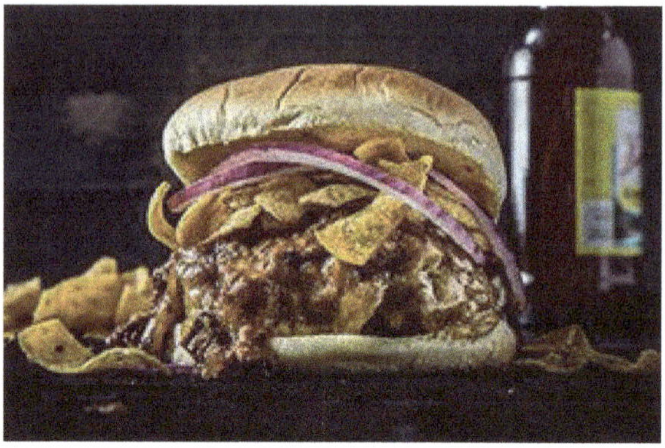

PREP TIME

20 MINS

COOK TIME

2.5 HRS

SERVES

4-6

HARDWOOD

HICKORY

INGREDIENTS

BEEF CHILI

2.5 LBS GROUND BEEF

1 LARGE ONION, DICED

1 TSP KOSHER SALT

1 CAN CHIPOTLES IN ADOBO, MINCED WITH SAUCE

1/4 CUP CHILI POWDER

1-1/2 TBSP CUMIN POWDER

3 CLOVES GARLIC, PEELED AND MINCED

1 JALAPEÑO PEPPER, MINCED

1 (14 OZ) CAN DICED OR CRUSHED TOMATOES

2 CUPS CHICKEN STOCK

1/8 CUP FLOUR

1/2 TBSP DARK CHILI POWDER

1/2 TBSP GROUND CINNAMON

JUICE OF 1 LIME

1 HERSHEY'S CHOCOLATE BAR

SALT AND PEPPER, TO TASTE

CHILI BURGERS

2 LBS GROUND BEEF

TRAEGER BEEF RUB, AS NEEDED

2 CUPS BEEF CHILI OR PREFERRED CHILI

5 HAMBURGER BUNS

5 SLICES CHEDDAR CHEESE

1 RED ONION, SLICED

1 BAG FRITO CORN CHIPS

PREPARATION

For the Beef Chili: Heat a large Dutch oven on the stove top over medium-high heat. Cook the ground beef until browned and cooked through.

Add all chili ingredients, minus the chocolate and limes to the Dutch oven.

When ready to cook, start the Traeger according to grill instructions. Set the temperature to 350 degrees F and preheat, lid closed for 10 to 15 minutes.

Put the Dutch oven into the grill for 2 hours, stirring every hour. Remove Dutch oven from grill.

Stir the lime juice and the chocolate into the chili. Set chili aside until ready to assemble the burgers.

For the burgers: When ready to cook, set the temperature to 350°F and preheat, lid closed for 15 minutes.

Form into 5 equal patties and season both sides with Traeger Beef Rub.

Place patties directly on the grill grate and cook for 4-5 minutes per side, flipping once. Top each burger with cheese and cook for 1 minute more to melt.

Remove from the grill and let rest 1-2 minutes.

To build burger, place the patty on the bottom bun, add a scoop of chili, Fritos, red onion and finish with the top bun. Enjoy!

TRAEGER FILET MIGNON

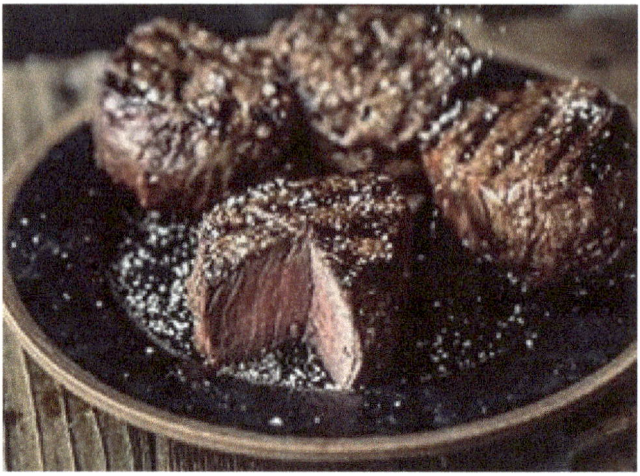

PREP TIME

5 MINS

COOK TIME

10 MINS

SERVES

2-4

HARDWOOD

HICKORY

INGREDIENTS

3 FILET MIGNON STEAKS

1 TSP SALT

1 TSP PEPPER

2 CLOVES GARLIC, MINCED

3 TBSP BUTTER, SOFTENED

PREPARATION

In a small bowl combine salt, pepper, garlic, and softened butter. Rub on both sides of filets. Let rest 10 minutes.

When ready to cook, set the temperature to 450°F and preheat, lid closed for 15 minutes.

Place steaks directly on the grill and cook for 5-8 minutes on each side, or until the filets reach an internal temperature of 135-140 degrees F for medium rare. Enjoy!

Pro Tip:

With filets there will not be much marbling, so look for a rich, red color.

WHISKEY BOURBON BBQ CHEESEBURGER

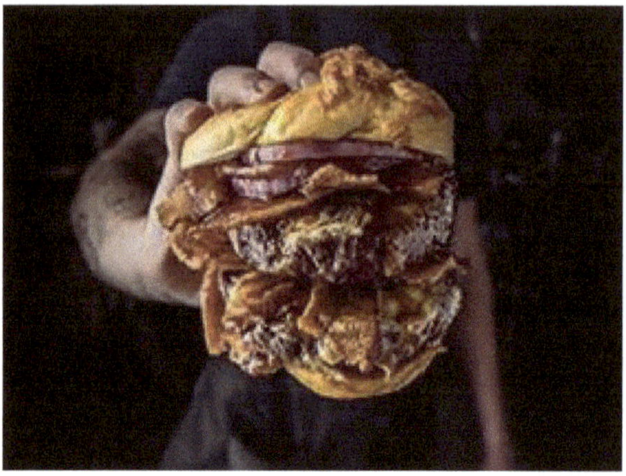

PREP TIME

20 MINS

COOK TIME

45 MINS

SERVES

4-6

HARDWOOD

HICKORY

INGREDIENTS

3 LBS GROUND BEEF

1/2 CUP BROWN SUGAR

HOT SAUCE TO TASTE

1/2 CUP WHISKEY BOURBON

TRAEGER RUB AS NEEDED

1 LB BACON

4 SLICES CHEDDAR CHEESE

1 RED ONION, SLICED

4 LARGE HAMBURGER BUNS

PREPARATION

In a medium bowl, combine ground beef and Traeger Rub and mix well using caution not to overwork or allow the beef to get too warm.

Divide the ground beef in quarters and put each quarter in a 6″ cake ring. Press down and form the beef into a patty.

With a skewer, poke about 40 holes about ¾″ of the way through each patty. Spread brown sugar all over the top of the patties then drizzle with hot sauce. Pour whisky over each burger, transfer to the fridge and let sit for about a half hour.

When ready to cook, set temperature to 225°F and preheat, lid closed for 10-15 minutes.

Remove burgers from the cake rings. When the grill is to temp, place bacon and burgers directly on the grill grate and cook until burgers internal temperature reaches 165 °F. In the last ten minutes of cooking, top with cheddar cheese to melt.

Remove burgers and bacon from the grill and build your burger to your liking. Enjoy!

STEAK TACO SALAD

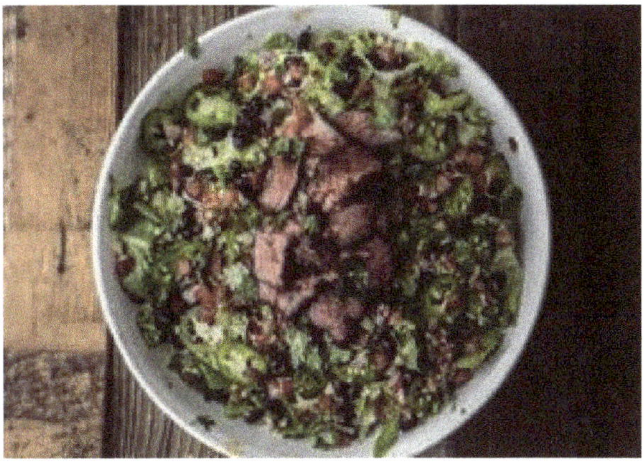

PREP TIME

15 MINS

COOK TIME

45 MINS

SERVES

4-6

HARDWOOD

HICKORY

INGREDIENTS

DRESSING

1 AVACADO

1 JALAPENO

1 EGG YOLK

1/2 BUNCH CILANTRO

1 CLOVE GARLIC

JUICE OF 1 LIME

1 CUP CANOLA OIL

SALAD

2- 8 OZ SNAKE RIVER FARM TOP SIRLOIN STEAKS

TRAEGER COFFEE RUB AS NEEDED

1 EAR OF CORN SHUCKED

1/2 TBSP OLIVE OIL

SALT TO TASTE

2 HEARTS ROMAINE

1 CAN BLACK BEANS, DRAINED AND RINSED

1/4 CUP PICO DE GALLO

1 JALAPENO, THINLY SLICED

1 TBSP CILANTRO LEAVES, TORN

PREPARATION

FOR THE DRESSING:

When ready to cook, set temperature to 180°F and preheat, lid closed for 15 minutes. For optimal flavor, use Super Smoke if available.

Cut the avocado in half and place it cut side up, directly on the grill grate. Smoke for 15-20 minutes until desired smoke flavor is achieved. Remove from grill and set aside to cool.

Scoop the flesh from the smoked avocado and place in the pitcher of a blender. Add remaining ingredients except for the oil and puree until smooth. With the motor running, gradually add the oil a little bit at a time until it has all been added and the mixture is emulsified. Season with salt and lime juice to taste.

FOR THE SALAD:

Season the steaks with Traeger coffee rub as needed. Brush the corn cob with olive oil and season with kosher salt.

When ready to cook set the temperature to 450 °F and preheat lid closed for 10-15 minutes.

Place the steaks and corn next to each other on the grill. Cook the steaks for about 5-7 minutes per side or until the internal temperature registers 130 °F for medium rare. Remove from grill and set aside to rest.

Allow the corn to cook for 15-20 minutes until the kernels are tender and the exterior is golden brown. This will take longer than the steaks to cook but should be done by the time the steaks have finished resting.

Chop the lettuce into bite sized pieces and place in a serving bowl. Toss with as much dressing as desired. Cut the kernels from the cob and sprinkle over the top of the dressed salad. Add black beans, pico, jalapeno, cilantro.

Thinly slice the steak and place on top of the salad. This salad, as is, is gluten free and dairy free but top with cheese if desired. Enjoy!

COWBOY CUT STEAK

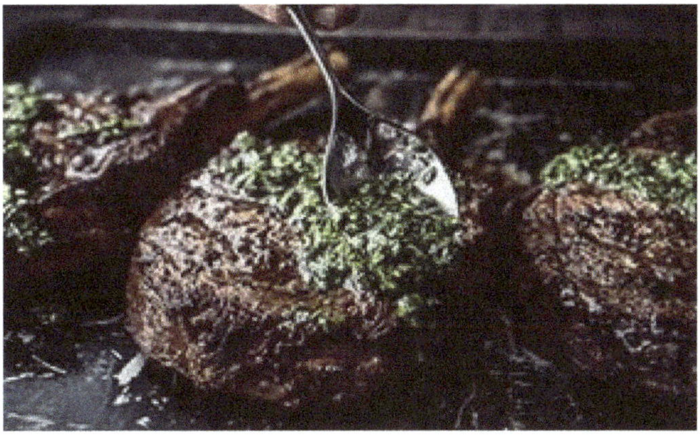

PREP TIME

10 MINS

COOK TIME

50 MINS

SERVES

4-6

HARDWOOD

MESQUITE

INGREDIENTS

STEAK

2 EA SNAKE RIVER FARMS COWBOY CUT STEAK (2.5 LBS EACH)

TRAEGER BEEF RUB TO TASTE

KOSHER SALT

GREMOLATA

1 BUNCH PARSLEY

2 TBSP CHOPPED MINT

1 TBSP PRESERVED LEMON, MINCED

1 CLOVE GARLIC MINCED

1/4 CUP OLIVE OIL

JUICE OF 1 LEMON

SALT AND PEPPER TO TASTE

PREPARATION

For the steaks:

Season the steaks liberally with Traeger Beef rub and kosher salt.

When ready to cook, set the temperature to 225 °F (with Super Smoke if using a WiFire enabled grill) and preheat lid closed for 10-15 minutes.

Place steaks directly on the grill grate and cook for 45 minutes or until the internal temperature reaches 115°F.

Remove steaks from the grill and let rest for 10 minutes.

While the steaks are resting, increase the grill temperature to high (450-500 °F) and preheat, lid closed for 10-15 minutes.

Place the steaks back on the grill and cook 5-7 minutes per side or until the internal reaches 130 °F for medium rare.

For the gremolata:

In a medium bowl combine all ingredients and stir well. Adjust seasoning to taste with salt and lemon juice.

Remove from the grill and let rest 1 minutes before slicing. Spoon gremolata over sliced steak to serve. Enjoy!

PORK RECIPES FOR WOOD PELLET SMOKER GRILL

THANKSGIVING SAUSAGE LEEK STUFFING

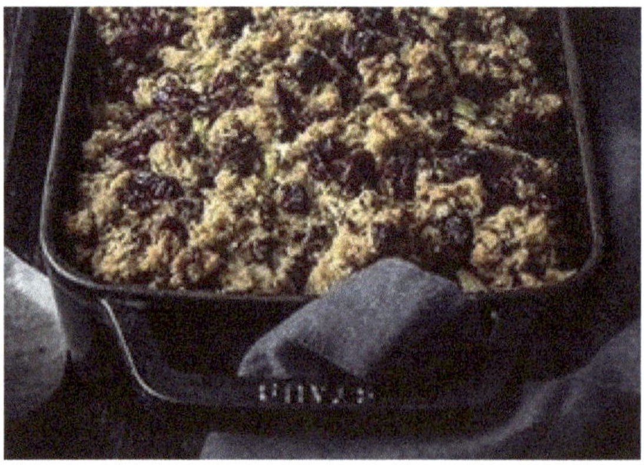

PREP TIME

10 MINS

COOK TIME

40 MINS

SERVES

8-12

HARDWOOD

MAPLE

INGREDIENTS

16 CUPS 1 INCH BREAD CUBES, WHITE, SOURDOUGH, OR CORN BREAD

1 STICK BUTTER

1 LEEK, THINLY SLICED

2 CUPS ONION, MEDIUM DICE

1 CUP CELERY, MEDIUM DICE

2 GRANNY SMITH APPLES, UNPEELED, CORED AND LARGE DICED

2 TBSP. FLAT-LEAF PARSLEY, CHOPPED

1 TBSP. KOSHER SALT

1 TSP. BLACK PEPPER, FRESHLY GROUND

1 LB. SWEET OR SPICY ITALIAN SAUSAGE, CASINGS REMOVED

2 CUPS CHICKEN STOCK, HOMEMADE PREFERABLY

1 CUP DRIED CRANBERRIES OR TOASTED PECANS (OPTIONAL)

PREPARATION

When ready to cook, set temperature to 300°F and preheat, lid closed for 15 minutes.

Place the bread cubes in a single layer on a sheet pan and bake for 7 minutes. Raise the Traeger temperature to 350°F. Remove the bread cubes to a very large bowl.

Meanwhile, in a large sauté pan, melt the butter and add the onions, celery, leeks, apples, parsley, salt and pepper. Sauté over medium heat for about 10 minutes or until the vegetables are softened. Add to the bread cubes.

In the same sauté pan, cook the sausage over medium heat for about 10 minutes, until browned and cooked through, breaking up the sausage with a fork while cooking. Add to the bread cubes and vegetables.

Add the chicken stock and cranberries or pecans to the mixture, mix well, and pour into a 9 by 12-inch baking dish. Bake for 30 minutes, until browned on top and hot in the middle. Serve warm.

SAGE & SAUSAGE STUFFING

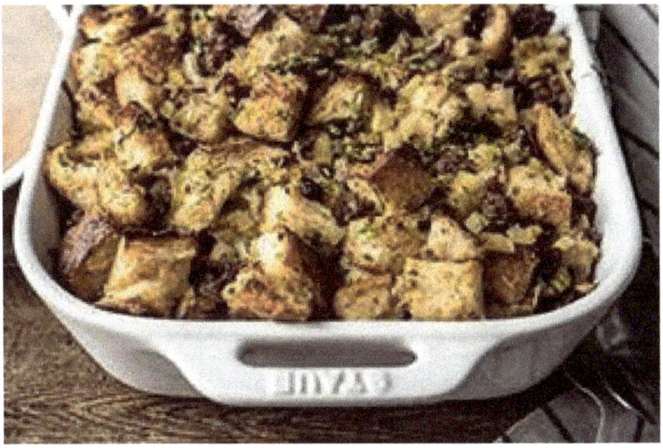

PREP TIME

20 MINS

COOK TIME

45 MINS

SERVES

4-6

HARDWOOD

MAPLE

INGREDIENTS

1 LB. SAGE-FLAVORED SAUSAGE, SUCH AS BOB EVANS OR JIMMY DEAN

1/2 CUP CELERY, DICED

1/2 CUP ONION, DICED

1 (14 OZ.) PACKAGE HERB-SEASONED STUFFING (SUCH AS PEPPERIDGE FARM)

2 TBSP. FRESH SAGE, CHOPPED

1 TBSP. FRESH THYME LEAVES OR MARJORAM, MINCED

1/2 CUP DRIED SWEETENED CRANBERRIES (OPTIONAL)

2 CUPS, PLUS MORE AS NEED TO MOISTEN THE STUFFING LOW-SODIUM CHICKEN BROTH

6 TBSP., PLUS MORE FOR GREASING THE BAKING DISH BUTTER

PREPARATION

Brown the sausage in a large frying pan, breaking up the sausage with a wooden spoon.

Add the onion and celery and cook until softened. Drain any excess fat. Transfer to a large mixing bowl. Add the stuffing mix, sage, thyme and cranberries, if using."

Warm the chicken broth over medium-low heat; add butter and cook until melted. Toss with the bread/sausage mixture and mix lightly.

Butter a 3-quart casserole or baking dish. Do not compress the mixture or it will be dense.

When ready to cook, set temperature to 350°F and preheat, lid closed for 15 minutes.

Bake the stuffing, covered, for 35 to 45 minutes; uncover during the last 20 minutes of cooking if you prefer a crunchier texture.

SMOKED PIG SHOTS RECIPE

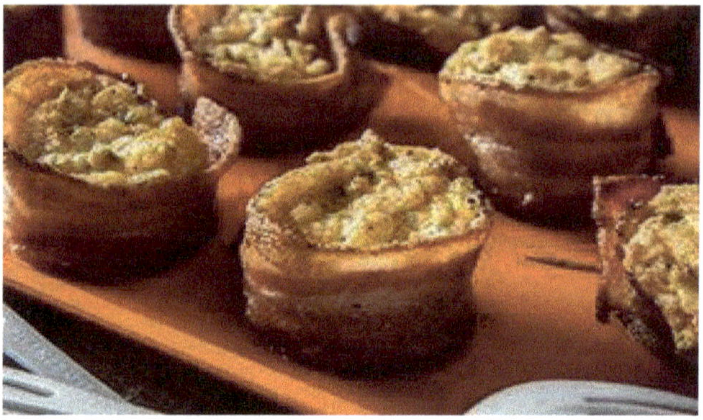

PREP TIME

10 MINS

COOK TIME

45 MINS

SERVES

8-12

HARDWOOD

HICKORY

INGREDIENTS

1 BLOCK CREAM CHEESE

2 LARGE GREEN CHILE PEPPERS, DICED (SUBSTITUTE 1 CAN DICED GREEN CHILES)

8 OZ CHEESE, SHREDDED

1 TBSP CHILI POWDER

2 TBSP MEAT CHURCH HONEY HOG

1 PACKAGE THICK CUT BACON

1 PACKAGE OF YOUR FAVORITE SMOKED SAUSAGE

TOOTHPICKS

PREPARATION

When ready to cook, start the Traeger grill on Smoke with the lid open until the fire is established (4 to 5 minutes). Set the temperature to 350 degrees F and preheat, lid closed, for 10 to 15 minutes.

Allow the cream cheese to soften. Mix cream cheese, chiles, shredded cheese, chili powder and Honey Hog thoroughly in a mixing bowl. Set aside. Slice sausage into 1/2-inch slices.

Cut bacon strips in half. Wrap bacon around the sausage, creating a bowl and secure with a toothpick.

Fill the bowl with the cream cheese mixture. Top with more Honey Hog BBQ rub.

Place the pig shots on the Traeger until the bacon is crispy and golden brown, about 45 to 60 minutes.

Remove the pig shots from the grill and cool for 10 minutes, cream cheese will be hot. Enjoy!

GRILLED GERMAN SAUSAGE WITH A SMOKY TRAEGER TWIST

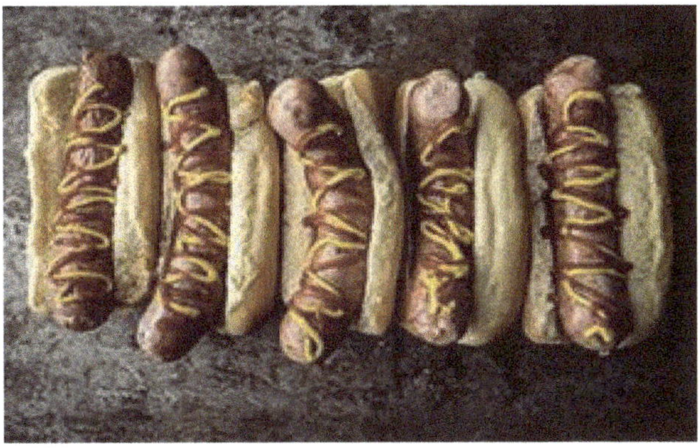

PREP TIME

20 MINS

COOK TIME

2 HRS

SERVES

8-12

HARDWOOD

HICKORY

INGREDIENTS

4 LBS GROUND PORK (80% LEAN 20% FAT)

1 LB GROUND VEAL OR GROUND BEEF

2 TBSP JACOBSEN SALT

1 TSP INSTACURE OR MORTON'S TENDERQUICK CURING SALT

1 TBSP GROUND NUTMEG

2 TSP GROUND MACE

1 TSP GROUND GINGER

1 CUP COLD MILK

2 EGGS

1 CUP NON-FAT DRY MILK POWDER

PREPARATION

Combine salt, tenderquick, nutmeg, mace and ginger in a large pitcher or small bowl.

Add the milk and eggs and beat until well combined. Pour the egg mixture over the ground meat and mix gently.

Using your hands, mix in the milk powder until evenly distributed.

Form the meat into sausage links.

When ready to cook, set the temperature to 450°F and preheat, lid closed for 15 minutes.

Smoke for approximately 2 hours or until the internal temperature reaches 175 degrees F.

Serve immediately or refrigerate until ready to serve. Enjoy!

PIZZA BITES

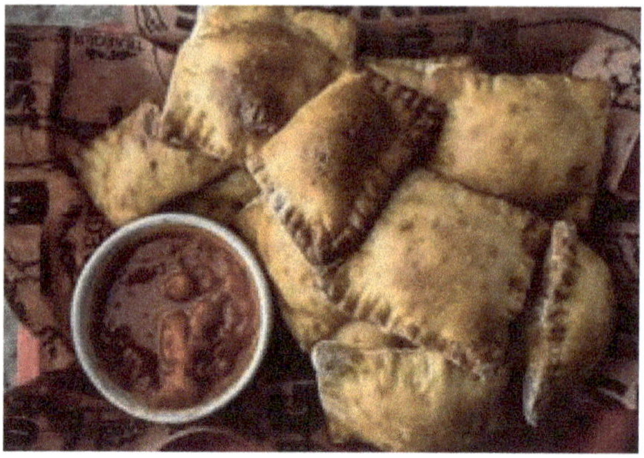

PREP TIME

24 HRS

COOK TIME

20 MINS

SERVES

6-8

HARDWOOD

MESQUITE

INGREDIENTS

PIZZA DOUGH

4 1/2 CUPS BREAD FLOUR, PLUS MORE FOR DUSTING

1 1/2 TBSP SUGAR

2 TSP INSTANT YEAST

3 TBSP EXTRA-VIRGIN OLIVE OIL

15 OZ LUKEWARM WATER

PIZZA FILLING

1 CUP MOZARELLA CHEESE

8 OZ PEPPERONI, CUT INTO THIN STRIPS

1 CUP PIZZA SAUCE

1 EGG FOR EGG WASH

PREPARATION

For the Pizza Dough: Combine flour, sugar, salt, and yeast in food processor. Pulse 3 to 4 times until incorporated evenly. Add olive oil and water. Run food processor until mixture forms ball that rides around the bowl above the blade, about 15 seconds. Continue processing 15 seconds longer.

Transfer dough ball to lightly floured surface and knead once or twice by hand until smooth ball is formed. Divide dough into three even parts and place each into a 1 gallon zip top bag. Place in refrigerator and allow to rise at least one day.

At least two hours before baking, remove dough from refrigerator and shape into balls by gathering dough towards bottom and pinching shut. Flour well and place each one in a separate medium mixing bowl. Cover tightly with plastic wrap and allow to rise at warm room temperature until roughly doubled in volume.

When ready to cook, set the temperature to 350°F and preheat, lid closed for 15 minutes.

After the first rise remove the dough from the fridge and let come to room temperature. Roll dough on a flat surface. Cut dough into long strips 3″ wide by 18″ long.

Slice pepperoni into strips.

In a medium bowl combine the pizza sauce, mozzarella and pepperoni.

Spoon 1 TBSP of the pizza filling onto the pizza dough every two inches, about halfway down the length of the dough. Dip a pastry brush into the egg wash and brush around pizza filling. Fold the half side of the dough (without the pizza filling) over the other the half that contains the pizza filling.

Press down between each pizza bite slightly with your fingers. With a ravioli or pizza cutter, cut around each filling- creating a rectangle shape and sealing the crust in.

Transfer each pizza bite onto a parchment lined cookie sheet. Cover with a kitchen towel and let them rise for 30 minutes.

When ready to cook, preheat the grill to 350 ℉ with the lid closed for 10-15 minutes.

Brush the bites with remaining egg wash, sprinkle with salt and place directly on the sheet tray. Bake 10-15 minutes until the exterior is golden brown.

Remove from grill and transfer to a serving dish. Serve with extra pizza sauce for dipping and enjoy!

BACON AND BROWN SUGAR WRAPPED LIL SMOKIES

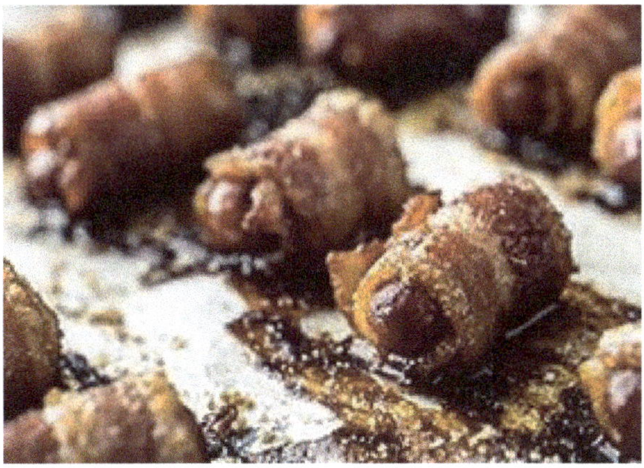

PREP TIME

20 MINS

COOK TIME

30 MINS

SERVES

6-8

HARDWOOD

APPLE

INGREDIENTS

1 PACKAGE (14 OZ) COCKTAIL SAUSAGES

1 LB BACON, STRIPS CUT IN HALF

1/2 CUP BROWN SUGAR

PREPARATION

Lay strips of bacon out on a clean flat surface. Roll out the bacon strips using a rolling pin, so they are a touch longer with even thickness.

Wrap each sausage in ½ strip of bacon and secure with a toothpick. Place the bacon wrapped sausages in a casserole dish in a single layer and cover with brown sugar. Transfer to the fridge and let sit for 30 minutes.

When ready to cook, set the temperature to 350°F and preheat, lid closed for 10-15 minutes.

Lay the sausages out on a parchment lined cookie sheet and place the sheet directly on the grill grate. Cook for 25-30 minutes until the bacon is crispy. Enjoy!

SMOKED MAPLE ICE CREAM WITH CANDIED BACON

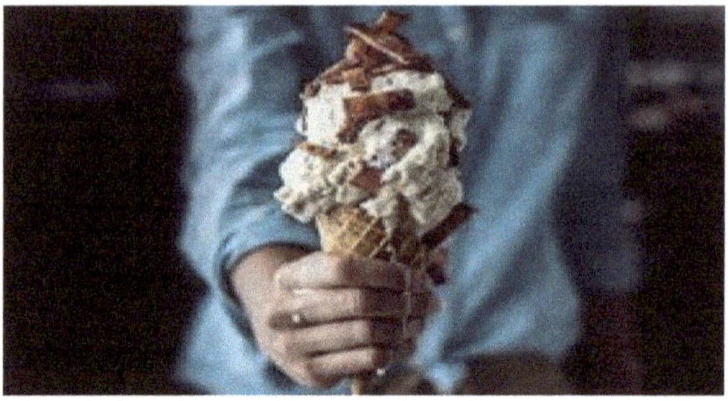

PREP TIME

20 MINS

COOK TIME

45 MINS

SERVES

4-6

HARDWOOD

MAPLE

INGREDIENTS

CANDIED BACON

8 SLICES BACON

1 TBSP PURE MAPLE SYRUP

1/4 CUP DARK BROWN SUGAR

ICE CREAM

2 CUPS HALF AND HALF

1 CUP HEAVY WHIPPING CREAM

1/3 CUP DARK BROWN SUGAR

1/3 CUP SUGAR

1/3 CUP MAPLE SYRUP

1 TSP VANILLA

1/2 TSP KOSHER SALT

1/4 TSP MAPLE FLAVORING

8-12 QUART SIZED ZIP TOP BAGS

5 LBS ICE

2 CUPS ICE CREAM SALT OR KOSHER SALT

PREPARATION

When ready to cook, set the temperature to 350°F and preheat, lid closed for 15 minutes.

In a small bowl, combine the 1/4 cup brown sugar and 1 tablespoon maple syrup to form a thick paste.

Spray a sheet pan with non-stick spray and then line with aluminum foil.

Lay the strips of bacon on the foil. Spread 1/2 tablespoon of the paste on each piece of bacon using the back of a spoon.

Place the sheet pan in the Traeger and cook for 15 minutes or until bacon is firm and glossy from the sugar.

Transfer the bacon to a cooling rack or plate and allow it to cool completely. When cooled, crumble bacon into a bowl and set aside.

Turn the heat on your Traeger down to Smoke.

In a 9x13 pan, combine all of the ingredients for the ice cream. Whisk until all of the sugar dissolves.

Place the pan in your Traeger and allow to smoke for 25-30 minutes, stirring occasionally.

Raise the temperature on your Traeger to 250 degrees F and, using a thermometer, cook until the temperature of your cream mixture reaches 170 degrees F, stirring occasionally. Do Not Exceed 170 Degrees, and do not allow your cream mixture to boil.

Take your cream mixture off the heat and allow to cool completely. Divide the cream mixture into 4-6 of the quart sized zip-top bags. Seal tightly and then insert those into a second bag and seal.

Fill a gallon zip-top bag with 1 pound of ice and 1/3 cup ice cream salt. Shake vigorously. Toss it back and forth.

Add ice and salt to the outer gallon bag as needed and drain the excess water.

When the ice cream mixture is frozen to your desired consistency, add in your bacon. Mix it directly into the ice cream or sprinkle on top. Enjoy!

TRAEGER BAKED CORN DOG BITES

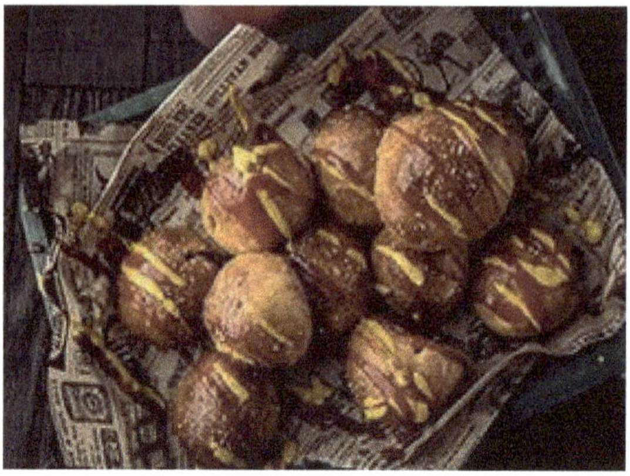

PREP TIME

45

COOK TIME

30

SERVES

10-12

HARDWOOD

HICKORY

INGREDIENTS

1 CUP MILK AT ROOM TEMP

4 TSP ACTIVE DRY YEAST

1/4 CUP GRANULATED SUGAR

2 CUPS ALL-PURPOSE FLOUR

1/2 CUP YELLOW CORN MEAL

1 TSP BAKING SODA

1/2 TSP MUSTARD POWDER

1/4 CUP VEGETABLE OIL

1/2 TSP CAYENNE PEPPER

1 EGG, LIGHTLY BEATEN

15 MINI HOT DOGS

1 TBSP DRIED MINCE GARLIC

1 TBSP COARSE SALT

KETCHUP & MUSTARD FOR SERVING

PREPARATION

When ready to cook, set the temperature to 375°F and preheat, lid closed for 15 minutes.

Combine milk, yeast and sugar in a bowl. Set aside for 5 minutes or until it starts to foam.

Then add oil, salt, cayenne pepper, mustard powder, baking soda, corn meal, all- purpose flour. Mix with a spoon until combined then use your hands to knead into a dough.

Transfer dough to a bowl and cover with plastic wrap and set aside for about 45 minutes- until dough rises and doubles in size.

Remove dough from bowl and divide into 15 pieces. On a working surface dusted with flour, use a rolling pin to roll out each piece of dough into 3″ x 3″ pieces. Place each hot dog in the middle of the sheet of dough. Roll it in the dough and press edges to seal to make 15 mini corn dog bites.

Transfer corn dog bites into a baking pan lined with parchment paper and brush each bite lightly with beaten egg. Sprinkle each bite with dried minced garlic and salt.

Bake in Traeger until golden brown- about 30 min.

Serve with ketchup and mustard or dipping sauce of your choice. Enjoy!

ST. LOUIS BBQ RIBS

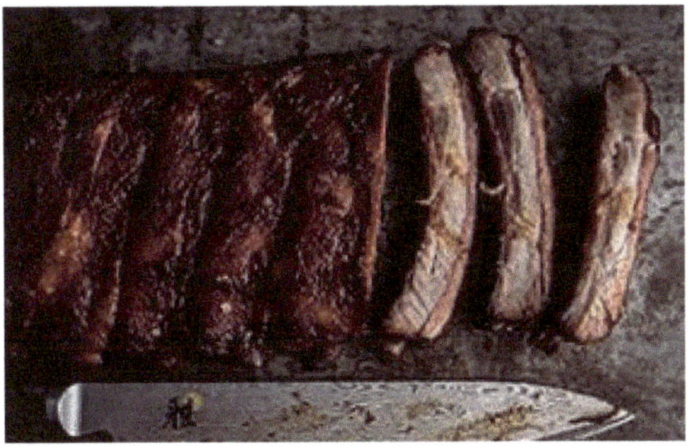

PREP TIME

20 MINS

COOK TIME

4 HRS

SERVES

4-6

HARDWOOD

PECAN

INGREDIENTS

2 RACKS ST. LOUIS BONE IN PORK RIBS

6 OZ TRAEGER PORK & POULTRY RUB

8 OZ APPLE JUICE

1 BOTTLE TRAEGER SWEET & HEAT BBQ SAUCE

PREPARATION

Trim ribs and peel off membrane from the back of ribs.

Apply an even coat of rub to the front and back of ribs. Let sit for 20 minutes and up to 4 hours if refrigerated.

When ready to cook, set temperature to 225°F and preheat, lid closed for 15 minutes.

Place ribs bone side down on grill grate. Put apple juice in a spray bottle and evenly spray ribs. Smoke for 1 hour.

After 1 hour, remove ribs from grill and wrap them in aluminum foil. Leave an opening at one end, pour in remainder of apple juice (about 6 oz) into the foil and wrap tightly.

Place ribs back on grill, meat side down and smoke for an additional 3 hours.

After 3 hours, start checking the internal temperature of ribs. Ribs are done when the internal temperature reaches 203°F.

When ribs are done, remove from the foil and brush a light layer of sauce on the front and back on the ribs. Return to the grill and cook an additional 10 minutes to set the sauce.

After sauce has set, take ribs off the grill and let rest for 10 minutes.

To serve, slice ribs in between the bones. Enjoy!

GRILLED LEMON PEPPER PORK TENDERLOIN

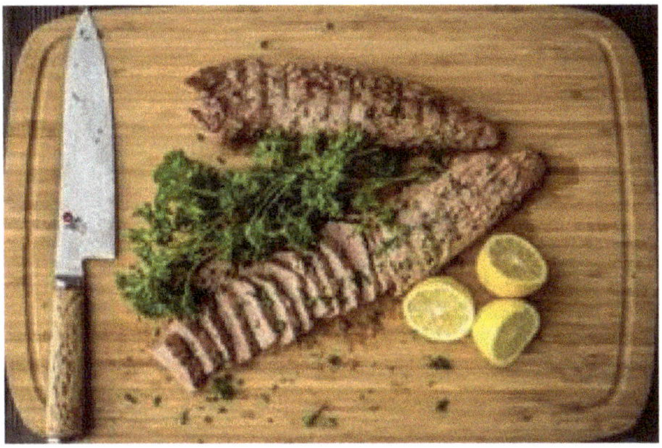

PREP TIME

20 MINS

COOK TIME

20 MINS

SERVES

4-6

HARDWOOD

APPLE

INGREDIENTS

ZEST OF 2 LEMONS

1 CLOVE GARLIC, MINCED

1 TSP FRESH PARSLEY, MINCED

1 TSP LEMON JUICE

1/4 TSP BLACK PEPPER

1/2 TSP KOSHER SALT

2 TBSP OLIVE OIL

1 (2 LB) PORK TENDERLOIN

PREPARATION

In a small bowl whisk together first 7 ingredients.

Trim all silverskin and excess fat from the tenderloin. Place in a large Ziploc bag. Pour the marinade over the tenderloin and zip closed.

Transfer to the refrigerator and marinate for at least 2 hours but no more than 8.

When ready to cook, set temperature to 375°F and preheat, lid closed for 15 minutes.

Remove the tenderloins from the bag and discard the marinade. When the grill is hot, place them directly on the grill grate and cook 15-20 minutes, flipping once halfway through until the internal temperature reaches 145°F.

Remove from the heat and let rest 5-10 minutes before slicing.

Enjoy!

LAMB RECIPES FOR WOOD PELLET SMOKER GRILLS

WHOLE RACK OF LAMB

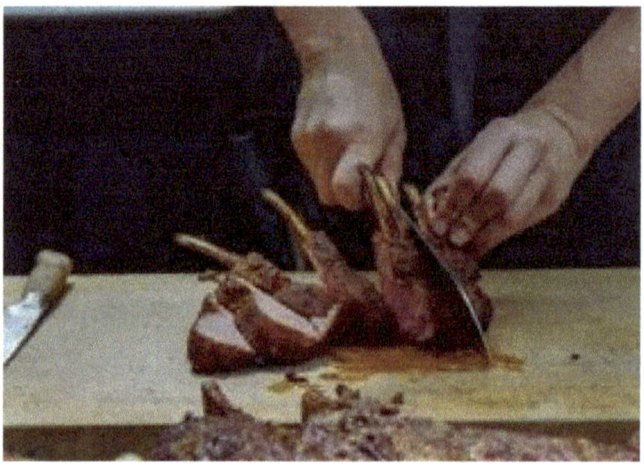

PREP TIME

10 MIN

COOK TIME

30 MIN

SERVES

4-6

HARDWOOD

HICKORY

INGREDIENTS

2 LB RACK OF GRASSFED LAMB

1 TBSP KOSHER SALT

8 CLOVES FRESH GARLIC

1 SMALL BUNCH FRESH THYME

2 TSP OLIVE OIL

1 TSP SHERRY VINEGAR

PREPARATION

Process the fresh garlic and all the thyme leaves in your food processor with the salt, oil and vinegar. Rub this pasted all over the rack of lamb.

When ready to cook, set the temperature to 450°F and prehcat, lid closed for 15 minutes

Lay the rack of lamb fat-side down on the grill and cook for 20 minutes. Turn over so the fat side is up and cook for an additional 10 minutes. Thermometer should be placed into the center of the lamb and should register 150-160°F.

Let rest for 10 minutes. Slice the rack into chops and serve. Enjoy!

SLOW ROASTED SHAWARMA

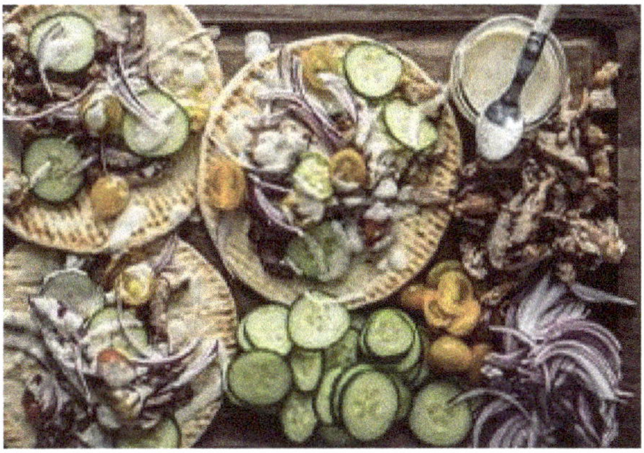

PREP TIME

25 MINS

COOK TIME

4.5 HRS

SERVES

6-8

HARDWOOD

MESQUITE

INGREDIENTS

5.5 LBS TOP SIRLOIN

5.5 LBS BONELESS SKINLESS CHICKEN THIGHS

4.5 LBS LAMB FAT

4 TBSP TRAEGER RUB

2 LARGE YELLOW ONIONS

PITA BREAD

TOPPING OPTIONS: CUCUMBER, TOMATOES, TAHINI, PICKLES, FRIES, ISRAELI SALAD

A DOUBLE SKEWER

A CAST IRON GRIDDLE

PREPARATION

*Plan ahead! Assemble the shawarma stack the night before you plan to cook it.

Slice all the meat and fat into ½" slices and place into 3 bowls (pro tip: it's easier to slice if they are all partially frozen).

Season each bowl with Traeger Rub and massage the rub into the meat.

Place half an onion on the bottom of each half skewer to make a firm base. then add 2 layers from each bowl at a time. Try to make the stack symmetrical, more or less. Then put the other 2 half onions at the top. Wrap in plastic wrap and refrigerate overnight.

When ready to cook, set temperature to 275°F and preheat, lid closed for 15 minutes.

Lay the shawarma directly on the grill grate and cook for about 3-4 hours, rotating at least once.

Remove from grill and increase the temperature to 445°F. While the grill preheats, place a cast iron griddle directly on the grill grate and brush with olive oil.

When the griddle is hot place the whole shawarma on the cast iron and sear 5-10 minutes per side. Remove from grill, slice off the edges, then repeat with remaining shawarma.

Serve in pita bread with your favorite toppings like cucumber, tomatoes, tahini, pickles, fries or Israeli salad.

Enjoy!

ROASTED LEG OF LAMB

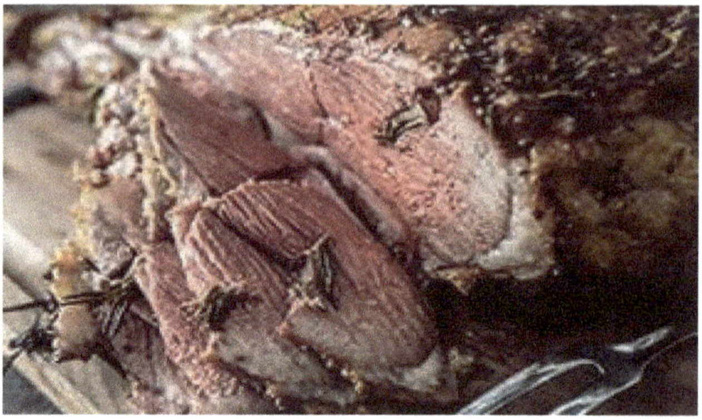

PREP TIME

30 MINS

COOK TIME

90 MINS

SERVES

8-12

HARDWOOD

CHERRY

INGREDIENTS

1 (7-8 LB) LEG OF LAMB, BONE-IN

1 TBSP GARLIC, CRUSHED

4 CLOVES GARLIC, SLICED LENGTHWISE

4 SPRIGS ROSEMARY, CUT INTO 1" PIECES

2 TSP OLIVE OIL

2 LEMONS

SALT AND PEPPER, TO TASTE

PREPARATION

Combine olive oil and the crushed garlic. Rub mixture on the leg of lamb.

With a paring knife, make small 3/4-inch deep perforations in the lamb, about 2 dozen. Stuff the slivered garlic and cut rosemary sprigs into the perforations.

Zest and juice the lemons, spreading the zest and juice evenly over the lamb. Season lamb with salt and pepper.

When ready to cook, set temperature to High and preheat, lid closed for 15 minutes.

Place the leg of lamb on the grill and cook for 30 minutes.

Reduce grill temperature to 350°F and cook until the internal temperature reaches 130°F for medium-rare, about 60-90 minutes.

Let the lamb rest for 15 minutes before carving. Enjoy!

GRILLED LAMB CHOPS WITH ROSEMARY SAUCE

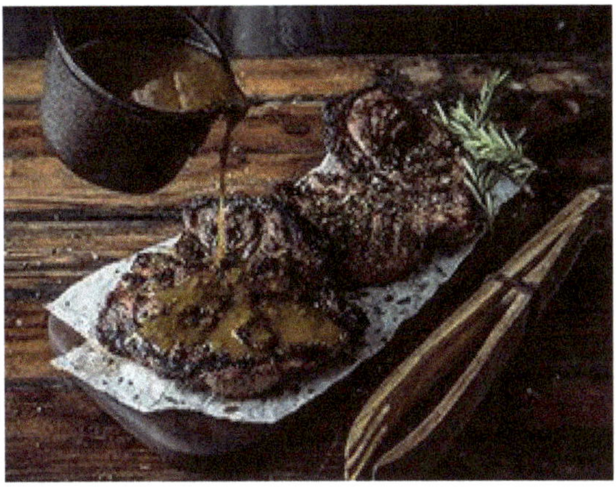

PREP TIME

15 MINS

COOK TIME

15 MINS

SERVES

6-8

HARDWOOD

APPLE

INGREDIENTS

1/2 CUP EXTRA VIRGIN OLIVE OIL, DIVIDED

1/4 CUP ONION OR SHALLLOT, COARSELY CHOPPED

2 CLOVES GARLIC, COARSELY CHOPPED

2 TBSP SOY SAUCE

2 TBSP BALSAMIC OR SHERRY VINEGAR

1 TBSP FRESH ROSEMARY NEEDLES

2 TSP DIJON MUSTARD

1 TSP WORCESTERSHIRE SAUCE

FRESHLY GROUND BLACK PEPPER, AS NEEDED

PREPARATION

In a small saucepan, sauté the onion and garlic in 1 tablespoon of olive oil over medium heat until softened and translucent. Do not let brown.

Transfer to a blender jar. Add the soy sauce, vinegar, rosemary, mustard, and Worcestershire and blend. Season to taste with black pepper.

Slowly drizzle in the remaining olive oil while the machine is running until the sauce is emulsified. Add a tablespoon of water if the sauce is too thick. Set aside.

When ready to cook, set temperature to High and preheat, lid closed for 15 minutes.

Brush the lamb chops on both sides with olive oil and season generously with salt and pepper.

Grill until lamb chops reach an internal temperature of 135°F for medium-rare, about 4 to 6 minutes per side.

Serve with the rosemary sauce for dipping. Enjoy!

ROASTED LEG OF LAMB WITH RED WINE REDUCTION

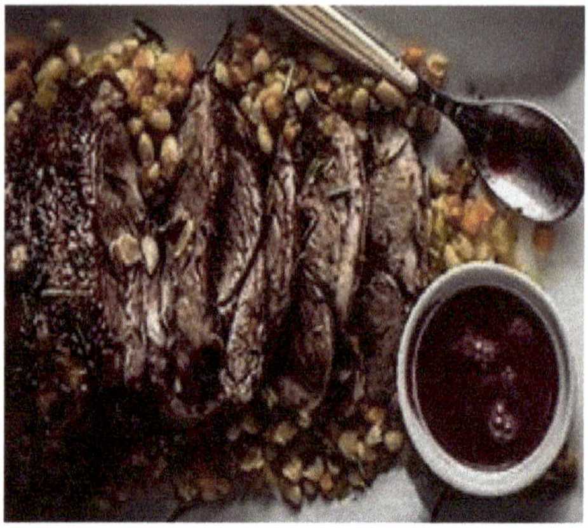

PREP TIME

4.5 HRS

COOK TIME

2 HRS

SERVES

8-12

HARDWOOD

APPLE

INGREDIENTS

1 (6-8 LB) BONE-IN LEG OF LAMB

10 GARLIC CLOVES, PEELED AND THINLY SLICED

3 TBSP ROSEMARY LEAVES, CHOPPED

2 TSP THYME LEAVES, CHOPPED

2 TBSP OLIVE OIL

1 TBSP KOSHER SALT

1/2 TSP FRESHLY GROUND PEPPER

1 CUP RED WINE

1 TSP KOSHER SALT

3 TBSP UNSALTED BUTTER

PREPARATION

Rinse lamb leg with water and pat dry. Using a sharp paring knife, create 20 1-inch slits all around the leg of lamb that are 1-inch deep. Place a sliver of garlic into each slit.

Combine the chopped rosemary and thyme with the olive oil, salt, and pepper. Using your hands, coat the lamb evenly with the herb oil.

Gently wrap lamb in saran wrap, place on a tray, and refrigerate for at least 4 hours to overnight. One hour before grilling, remove the lamb from the refrigerator.

Remove the plastic wrap and place the lamb on a roasting rack above a large roasting pan. Pour the red wine and stock into the bottom of the pan, ensuring the liquid does not touch the meat. If it is close, only use half of the wine and stock.

When ready to cook, set the temperature to High and preheat, lid closed for 15 minutes.

Place the lamb in its roasting pan directly on the grill grate and roast for 20 minutes. Reduce the heat to 350°F and roast another hour or more, about 10 to 12 minutes per pound or until the temperature reaches 130°F when a meat thermometer is inserted into the thickest part of the leg away from the bone.

Remove the meat from the grill and loosely tent with foil on a cutting board. Allow to rest for 15-20 minutes.

Meanwhile strain the juices from the pan into a medium saucepan removing any excess fat that has dropped into the pan.

Bring the juices to a boil, reduce to a simmer, and cook until it can coat the back of a spoon, about 10 minutes.

Whisk in the butter and taste, adding more salt and pepper as needed.

Carve the lamb and serve with the red wine jus. Enjoy!

GRILLED LAMB BURGERS WITH PICKLED ONIONS

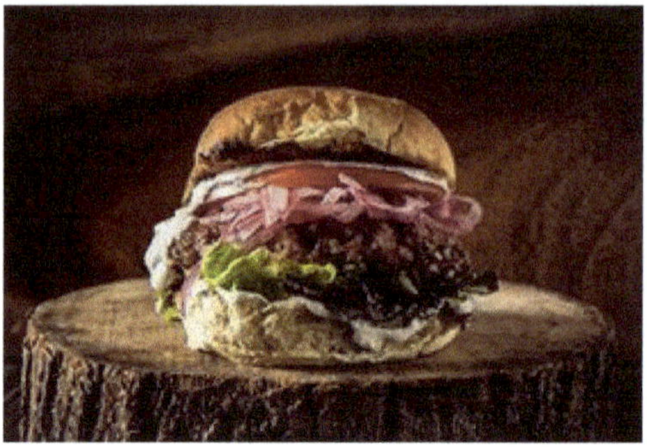

PREP TIME

10 MINS

COOK TIME

10 MINS

SERVES

4-6

HARDWOOD

HICKORY

INGREDIENTS

PICKLED ONIONS

1/2 RED ONION, THINLY SLICED

6 TBSP LIME JUICE

1/2 TSP KOSHER SALT

1/2 TSP RAW CANE SUGAR

YOGURT SAUCE

1 CUP GREEK YOGURT

2 TBSP LEMON JUICE

1 GARLIC CLOVE, MINCED

2 TBSP FINELY CHOPPED HERBS, SUCH AS MINT, DILL AND PARSLEY

1/2 TSP KOSHER SALT

LAMB BURGERS

1 TBSP OLIVE OIL

1/2 RED ONION, FINELY DICED

1 LB GROUND LAMB

8 OZ GROUND PORK

3 TBSP FINELY CHOPPED MINT

2 TBSP FINELY CHOPPED DILL

3 TBSP FINELY CHOPPED PARSLEY

4 GARLIC CLOVES, MINCED

1 1/2 TSP GROUND CUMIN

1 TSP GROUND CORIANDER

1 TSP KOSHER SALT

1/2 TSP FRESHLY GROUND BLACK PEPPER

1 SLICED TOMATO

6 BUNS

SLICED CUCUMBER

BUTTER LETTUCE

PREPARATION

To Pickle the Onions: Place the onion, lime juice, salt and sugar in a small bowl. Stir to combine, cover and let sit at room temperature for about 2 hours to soften. Refrigerate until ready to use.

To make the Yogurt Sauce: In a small bowl, stir together the yogurt, lemon juice, garlic, herbs, and 1/2 tsp salt. Adjust the salt to taste. Cover and refrigerate until ready to serve, or for up to 2 days.

To make the lamb burgers: In a small skillet over medium heat, warm the olive oil. Add the onion and cook, stirring frequently until softened, about 7 minutes. Transfer to a small plate to cool.

In a large bowl, combine the lamb, pork, mint, dill, parsley, garlic, cumin, coriander, salt, pepper, and cooled onions. Gently mix with your hands. Do not overwork the meat.

Divide the mixture into 6 equal balls. Press into patties and transfer to a parchment-lined baking sheet. If not cooking immediately, cover and refrigerate for up to 8 hours.

When ready to cook, set the temperature to High and preheat, lid closed for 15 minutes.

Place the burgers on the grill and cook until well-browned, about 2 to 3 minutes per side for medium-rare, or about 5 minutes per side for well done.

Transfer burgers to a plate to rest for 5 minutes before serving.

Place burgers on buns and top with a generous dollop of herbed yogurt sauce and some pickled onions.

Add lettuce, sliced tomatoes or cucumbers if desired. Serve immediately. Enjoy!

BRAISED LAMB SHANK

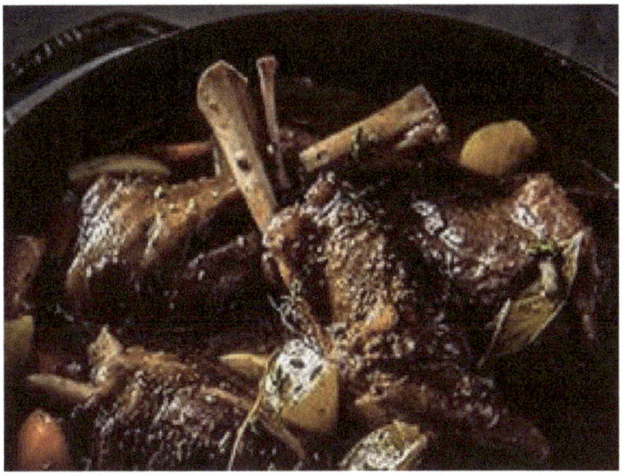

PREP TIME

15 MINS

COOK TIME

4 HRS

SERVES

4-6

HARDWOOD

MESQUITE

INGREDIENTS

4 SHANKS LAMB

OLIVE OIL, AS NEEDED

TRAEGER PRIME RIB RUB

1 CUP BEEF BROTH

1 CUP RED WINE

4 SPRIGS FRESH ROSEMARY AND THYME

PREPARATION

Season the lamb shanks liberally with Traeger Prime Rib Rub.

When ready to cook, set the temperature to High and preheat, lid closed for 15 minutes.

Place the shanks directly on the grill grate and cook for 20 minutes or until the exterior has browned.

Transfer the shanks to a dutch oven and pour in beef broth, wine, and add herbs. Cover with a tight fitting lid and place back on the grill grate reducing the temperature to 325°F.

Braise the shanks for 3-4 hours until the internal temperature is 180°F. Take care not to touch bone with the tip of the temperature probe or you will get a false reading.

Carefully lift the lid and transfer the lamb and any accumulated juices to a platter or plates. Enjoy!

GREEK STYLE ROAST LEG OF LAMB RECIPE

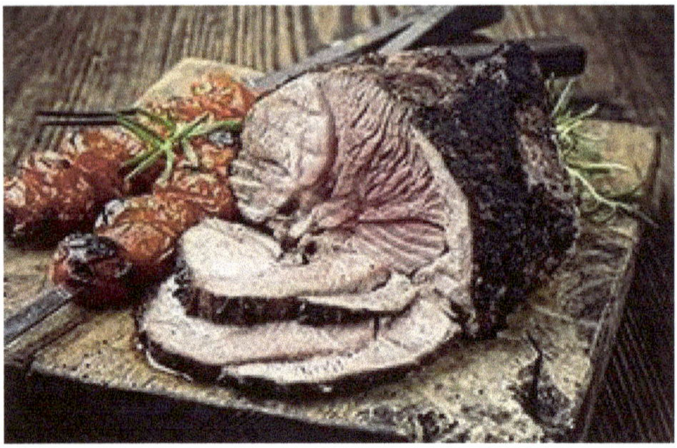

PREP TIME

25 MINS

COOK TIME

1.5 HRS

SERVES

8-12

HARDWOOD

OAK

INGREDIENTS

ONE 6-7 LBS. LEG OF LAMB, BONE-IN

8 CLOVES GARLIC

2 SPRIGS FRESH ROSEMARY, NEEDLES STRIPPED, STEMS DISCARDED

1 SPRIG (OR 1 TSP. DRIED) FRESH OREGANO

2 LEMONS, JUICED

6 TBSP. EVOO (EXTRA-VIRGIN OLIVE OIL)

AS NEEDED COARSE SALT (KOSHER) AND BLACK PEPPER, FRESHLY GROUND

PREPARATION

Using a paring knife, make a series of small slits in the leg.

On a cutting board, finely mince the garlic, rosemary, and oregano with a chef's knife to make an herb and garlic paste. (Alternatively, put the garlic and herbs in a small food processor.)

Stuff a small amount of the paste into each of the slits, driving it into the slit with a spoon handle or other utensil. Put the lamb on a rack inside a roasting pan. If desired, like the pan with foil for easier clean-up.

Rub the outside of the lamb with the lemon juice, then the olive oil. Cover with plastic wrap and refrigerate for at least 8 hours, or overnight.

Remove from the refrigerator and let the lamb come to room temperature.

Remove the plastic wrap and season the lamb with salt and pepper. When ready to cook, start the Traeger grill on Smoke with the lid open until the fire is established (4 to 5 minutes). Set the temperature to 400F and preheat, lid closed, for 10 to 15 minutes.

Roast the lamb for 30 minutes. Reduce the heat to 350F (300 if you have a manual controller) and continue to cook until the internal temperature in the thickest part of the meat - be sure the temperature probe is not touching bone - is about 140F for medium-rare, about 1 hour more, longer if you're cooking at 300F or prefer your lamb more well-done.

Transfer the lamb to a cutting board and let rest for 15 minutes before slicing on a diagonal into thin slices.

SMOKED LAMB SAUSAGE

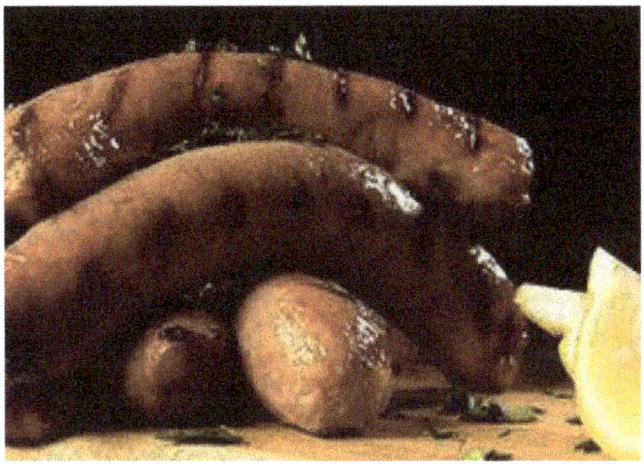

PREP TIME

60 MINS

COOK TIME

70 MINS

SERVES

6-8

HARDWOOD

CHERRY

INGREDIENTS

SMOKED LAMB SAUSAGE

2 LB. LAMB SHOULDER

1 QTY. (60 INCH) HOG CASING

1 TBSP. GARLIC

1 TSP. CUMIN

1 TSP. PAPRIKA

1/2 TSP. CAYENNE

2 TBSP. GROUND FENNEL

1 TBSP. CILANTRO, FINELY CHOPPED

1 TBSP. PARSLEY, FINELY CHOPPED

1 TSP. BLACK PEPPER

2 TBSP. SALT

SAUCE

3 CUPS GREEK YOGURT

1 LEMON, JUICED

1 CLOVE GARLIC

1 CUCUMBER, PEELED, SHREDDED, AND DRAINED

1 TBSP. DILL

TO TASTE SALT & PEPPER

PREPARATION

Cut the lamb shoulder into 2-inch pieces, and using a meat grinder, grind the meat.

Lightly combine the lamb with all the spices in a bowl and refrigerate. It is important to refrigerate the ground lamb so the fat does not melt in order to give the sausage a good texture.

Next, using a sausage horn, attach the hog casing and start to feed the sausage back through the grinder to fill the casing and twist into links. With a paring knife, prick holes all along the casing (this will allow steam to escape while cooking). Refrigerate.

Combine all ingredients for the yogurt sauce in a medium sized bowl. Cover and refrigerate.

When ready to cook, start your Traeger on Smoke, with the lid open until the fire is established (4 to 5 minutes). Set the temperature to 225°F, place the prepared sausage on the grill grate and smoke it for 1 hour.

Once the hour is up, remove the links from the grill and turn the grill up to High (450°F) and preheat (10-15 minutes). Once the grill has reached 450°F, place the links back on the grill and cook for 5 minutes on each side.

Serve hot with yogurt sauce and roasted potatoes on the side. Enjoy!

LAMB LOLLIPOPS WITH MANGO CHUTNEY

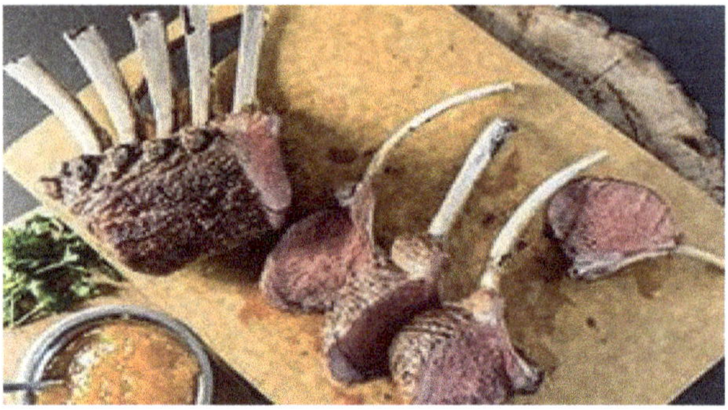

PREP TIME

15 MINS

COOK TIME

10 MINS

SERVES

4-6

HARDWOOD

APPLE

INGREDIENTS

LAMB LOLLIPOPS

6 LAMB CHOPS, AROUND 3/4-INCH-THICK, FRENCHED

2 TBSP OLIVE OIL

1/2 TSP COURSE KOSHER SALT

1/2 TSP BLACK PEPPER, FRESHLY CRACKED

2 TBSP FRESH MINT, CHOPPED

MANGO CHUTNEY

1 MANGO, PEELED, SEEDED AND CHOPPED

3 CLOVES GARLIC, CHOPPED

1/2 HABANERO PEPPER, SEEDED AND CHOPPED, OR MORE TO TASTE

3 SPRIGS FRESH CILANTRO, CHOPPED

1 TBSP FRESH LIME JUICE

1 TEASPOON SALT

1/2 TSP PEPPER, FRESHLY CRACKED

PREPARATION

If you can't purchase frenched lamb chops, using a sharp knife, cut and scrape the flesh and fat off the bone to make it look like a lollipop.

Add all chutney ingredients into a food processor and pulse about 15 times or until desired consistency; set aside. Chop mint and set aside.

When ready to cook, start the Traeger grill on Smoke with the lid open until the fire is established (4 to 5 minutes). Set the temperature to High and preheat, lid closed, for 10 to 15 minutes.

While grill preheats, on a baking sheet drizzle lamb lollipops with olive. Coat both sides. Season both sides with salt and pepper and allow to sit at room temperature for 5 to 10 minutes.

Place the lamb pops directly on grill grate. Close lid and grill for 5 minutes. Flip over and grill for another 3 minutes or until a thermometer inserted into the thickest part of the meat registers an internal temperature of 130 degrees F.

Remove from grill and allow to rest 10 minutes before serving.

Spoon chutney over each lamb lollipop and sprinkle with fresh chopped mint. Enjoy!

VEGETABLES RECIPES FOR WOOD PELLET SMOKER GRILLS

BAKED GREEN BEAN CASSEROLE

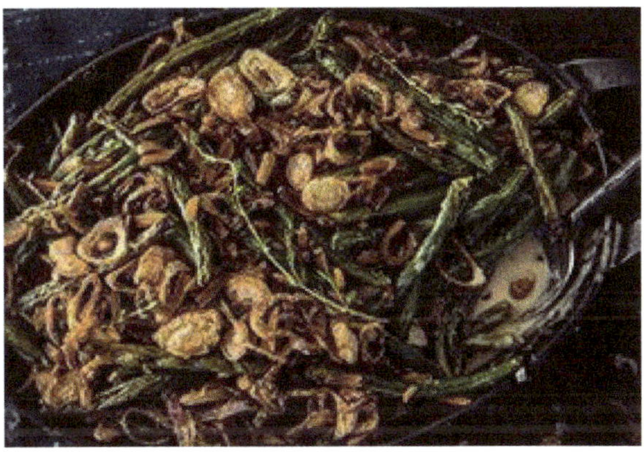

PREP TIME

10 MINS

COOK TIME

50 MINS

SERVES

10-12

HARDWOOD

PECAN

INGREDIENTS

3 LBS TRIMMED GREEN BEANS

KOSHER SALT

2 TBSP OLIVE OIL

2 TBSP UNSALTED BUTTER

1/2 LB SHITAKE OR KING TRUMPET MUSHROOMS, SLICED

1/4 CUP MINCED SHALLOT

1/4 CUP RICE FLOUR

2 CUPS CHICKEN STOCK

1/2 CUP SHERRY COOKING WINE

1 CUP HEAVY CREAM

1 CUP GRATED PARMIGIANO REGGIANO

1 CUP SLIVERED ALMONDS, FOR TOPPING

4 CUPS CANOLA OR VEGETABLE OIL

8 WHOLE, PEELED SHALLOTS

1/2 CUP RICE FLOUR

1 TSP KOSHER SALT

PREPARATION

When ready to cook, set the temperature to High and preheat, lid closed for 15 minutes.

Fill a large stockpot 2/3 full with water and bring to a boil over high heat. Prepare a large ice bath. When the water is boiling, add 1 Tbsp of salt.

After the water has returned to a rolling boil, add half of the green beans. Cook until al dente, about 2 minutes. Remove with a strainer and place the beans in the ice bath to cool.

Remove the green beans from the water and place on paper towels to dry. Repeat with the remaining green beans. Alternatively, place the green beans on a clean dish cloth and roll up to remove the water.

To make the Sauce: Melt the butter and olive oil in a small saucepan over medium heat. Add the shallots and mushrooms and a generous pinch of salt and cook, stirring, until the mushrooms are soft, about 5 minutes.

Sprinkle the rice flour over the top and stir to coat the mushrooms and cook off the raw flour taste, about 2 minutes. Add the sherry, stir and reduce, then slowly stir in the stock, allowing to thicken and ensuring there are no lumps, about 3 minutes.

Stir in the cream and Parmigiano-Reggiano. Taste, adding salt and pepper as needed.

Combine the green beans with the sauce. Pour into a large serving dish that is oven-proof. Sprinkle with almonds. Bake on the Traeger until the sauce is bubbling and the almonds are browned, about 30 minutes.

While the green beans are on the grill, fry the shallots. Place the oil in a deep saucepan or Dutch oven and heat oil to 350°F.

Combine the rice flour and salt in a shallow bowl and mix with a fork. Slice the shallots into 1/8-inch rings. Toss the shallots to coat in the rice flour, shaking off any excess in a sieve.

Fry the shallots in batches until golden brown, about 30 seconds to one minute. Drain on paper towels.

When the casserole is ready, garnish with the fried shallots. Enjoy!

MASHED POTATOES

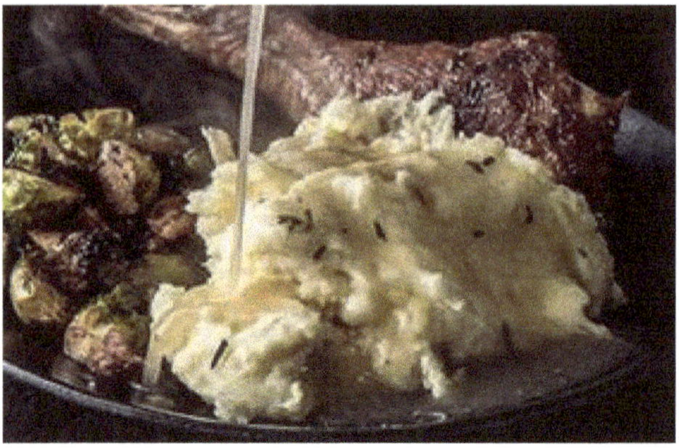

PREP TIME

5 MINS

COOK TIME

40 MINS

SERVES

8-12

HARDWOOD

HICKORY

INGREDIENTS

5 LBS YUKON GOLD POTATOES, LARGE DICE

1 1/2 STICKS BUTTER, SOFTENED

1 1/2 CUP CREAM, ROOM TEMPERATURE

KOSHER SALT, TO TASTE

WHITE PEPPER, TO TASTE

PREPARATION

When ready to cook, set temperature to 300°F and preheat, lid closed for 15 minutes

Peel and dice potatoes into 1/2" cubes.

Place the potatoes in a foil tin and cover. Roast in the Traeger until tender (about 40 minutes).

In a medium sauce pan, combine cream and butter. Cook over medium heat until butter is melted.

Mash potatoes using a potato masher. Gradually add in cream and butter mixture, and mix using the masher. Be careful not to overwork, or the potatoes will becomes gluey.

Season with salt and pepper to taste. Enjoy!

CORN & CHEESE CHILE RELLENOS

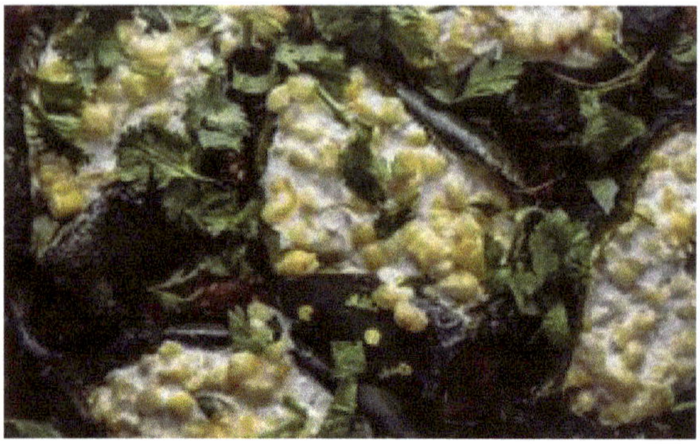

PREP TIME

30 MINS

COOK TIME

65 MINS

SERVES

8-12

HARDWOOD

MAPLE

INGREDIENTS

2 LBS. RIPE TOMATOES, CHOPPED

4 CLOVES GARLIC, CHOPPED

1/2 CUP SWEET ONION, CHOPPED

1 JALAPENO, STEMMED, SEEDED, AND CHOPPED

8 LARGE GREEN NEW MEXICAN OR POBLANO CHILES

3 EARS SWEET CORN, HUSKED

1/2 TSP. DRY OREGANO, MEXICAN, CRUMBLED

1 TSP. GROUND CUMIN

1 TSP. MILD CHILE POWDER

1/8 TSP. GROUND CINNAMON

SALT AND FRESHLY GROUND PEPPER

3 CUPS GRATED MONTEREY JACK

1/2 CUP MEXICAN CREMA

1 CUP QUESO FRESCO, CRUMBLED

FRESH CILANTRO LEAVES

PREPARATION

Put the tomatoes, garlic, onion, and jalapeno in a shallow baking dish and place on the grill grate before starting your Traeger. (This will expose the vegetables to more wood smoke.)

When ready to cook, start the Traeger grill on Smoke with the lid open until the fire is established (4 to 5 minutes). Set the temperature to 450F and preheat, lid closed, for 10 to 15 minutes.

When the grill is hot, arrange the New Mexican chiles and the sweet corn on the grate and grill until the chiles are blistered and blackened in spots and the corn is lightly browned, 15 to 20 minutes for the chiles and 10 to 15 minutes for the corn, turning with tongs as needed.

Stir the tomato-onion mixture once or twice and remove it from the grill grate when the tomatoes begin to break down. Let all the vegetables cool.

Reduce the heat of the Traeger to 350F if you intend to bake the rellenos right away. (You can also make the sauce and assemble the rellenos the day before you bake them. Cover and refrigerate.)

Put the cooled tomato mixture in a blender and liquefy. Pour into a saucepan.

Stir in the cumin, oregano, chile powder, cinnamon, and salt and pepper to taste. Simmer over medium heat for 15 to 20 minutes, or until the sauce is slightly thickened, stirring occasionally.

Carefully peel the blistered outer skin off the New Mexican chiles: Leave the stem ends intact, and try not to tear the flesh.

With a small paring knife, slit each chile lengthwise from the shoulder (just below the stem) to the tip. Pull out the seeds and set the chiles aside while you make the filling.

Slice the corn off the cobs and put in a large mixing bowl. Toss with 2 cups of the cheese, reserving 1 cup. Gently stir in the sour cream. Season with salt and pepper. Generously stuff the chiles with the corn-cheese mixture and arrange shoulder to shoulder, cut sides up, in a baking dish or on a rimmed baking sheet. (Line with foil for easy clean-up, if desired.) Sprinkle some of the reserved cheese on top of each relleno.

Bake the rellenos for 25 to 30 minutes, or until the filling is bubbling and the cheese has melted. Reheat the tomato sauce if necessary.

To serve, put a small pool of tomato sauce on each plate and arrange a relleno in the center of it. Sprinkle with queso fresco and garnish with fresh cilantro leaves, if desired. Enjoy!

ROASTED TOMATOES WITH HOT PEPPER SAUCE

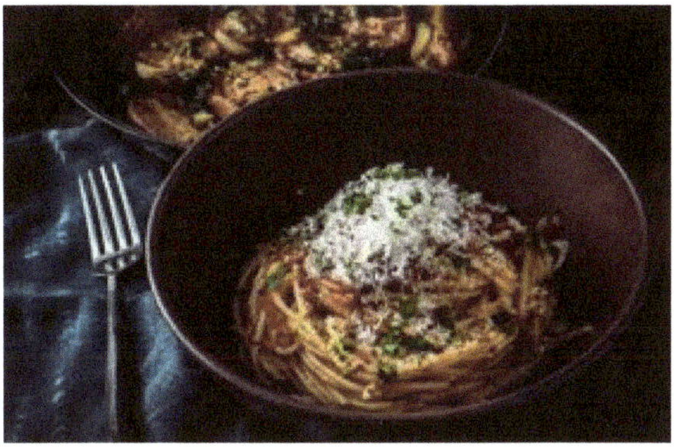

PREP TIME

20 MINS

COOK TIME

90 MINS

SERVES

4-6

HARDWOOD

ALDER

INGREDIENTS

2 LBS ROMA FRESH TOMATOES

3 TBSP PARSLEY, CHOPPED

2 TBSP GARLIC, CHOPPED

BLACK PEPPER, TO TASTE

1/2 CUP OLIVE OIL

HOT PEPPER, TO TASTE

1 LB SPAGHETTI OR OTHER PASTA

PREPARATION

When ready to cook, set the temperature to 400°F and preheat, lid closed for 15 minutes

Wash tomatoes and cut them in half, length width. Place them in a baking dish cut side up.

Sprinkle with chopped parsley, garlic, add salt and black pepper and pour 1/4 cup of olive oil over them.

Place on pre-heated Traeger and bake for 1 1/2 hours. Tomatoes will shrink and the skins will be partly blackened.

Remove tomatoes from baking dish and place in a food processor leaving the cooked oil, and puree them.

Drop pasta into boiling salted water and cook until tender. Drain and toss immediately with the pureed tomatoes.

Add the remaining 1/4 cup of raw olive oil and crumbled hot red pepper to taste. Toss and serve. Enjoy!

GRILLED FINGERLING POTATO SALAD

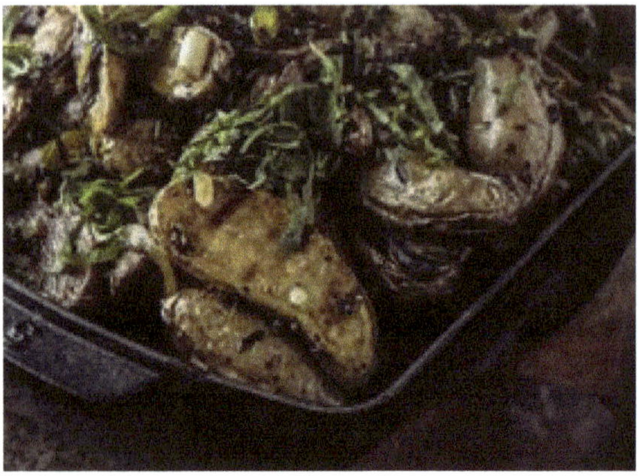

PREP TIME

15 MINS

COOK TIME

15 MINS

SERVES

6-8

HARDWOOD

PECAN

INGREDIENTS

1-1/2 LBS. FINGERLING POTATOES CUT IN HALF LENGTHWISE

10 SCALLIONS

2/3 CUP EVOO (EXTRA VIRGIN OLIVE OIL), DIVIDED USE

2 TBSP RICE VINEGAR

2 TSP LEMON JUICE

1 SMALL JALAPENO, SLICED

2 TSP KOSHER SALT

PREPARATION

When ready to cook, set temperature to High and preheat, lid closed for 15 minutes.

Brush the scallions with the oil and place on the grill. Cook until lightly charred, about 2-3 minutes. Remove and let cool. Once the scallions have cooled, slice and set aside.

Brush the Fingerlings with oil (reserving 1/3 cup for later use), then salt and pepper. Place cut side down on the grill until cooked through, about 4-5 minutes.

In a bowl, whisk the remaining 1/3 cup olive oil, rice vinegar, salt, and lemon juice, then mix in the scallions, potatoes, and sliced jalapeo.

Season with salt and pepper, and serve. Enjoy!

SMOKED JALAPEÑO POPPERS

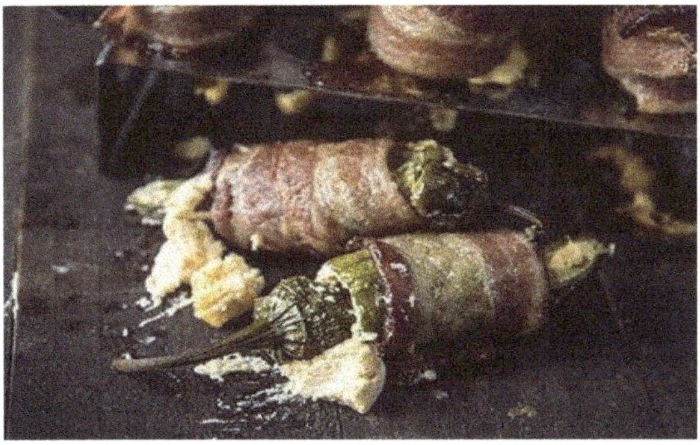

PREP TIME

15 MINS

COOK TIME

60 MINS

SERVES

4-6

HARDWOOD

MESQUITE

INGREDIENTS

12 MEDIUM JALAPEÑOS

6 SLICES BACON, CUT IN HALF

8 OZ CREAM CHEESE, SOFTENED

1 CUP CHEESE, GRATED

2 TBSP TRAEGER PORK & POULTRY RUB

PREPARATION

When ready to cook, set temperature to 180°F and preheat, lid closed for 15 minutes.

Slice the jalapeños in half lengthwise. Scrape out any seeds and ribs with a small spoon or paring knife.

Mix softened cream cheese with Traeger Pork & Poultry rub and grated cheese.

Spoon mixture onto each jalapeño half. Wrap with bacon and secure with a toothpick.

Place the jalapeños on a rimmed baking sheet. Place on grill and smoke for 30 minutes.

Increase the grill temperature to 375°F and cook an additional 30 minutes or until bacon is cooked to desired doneness. Serve warm, enjoy!

GRILLED VEGGIE SANDWICH

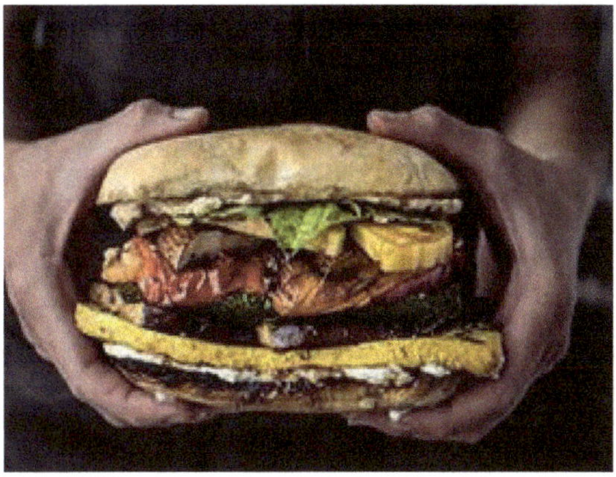

PREP TIME

30 MINS

COOK TIME

30 MINS

SERVES

4-6

HARDWOOD

PECAN

INGREDIENTS

SMOKED HUMMUS

1-1/2 CUPS CHICKPEAS

1/3 CUP TAHINI

1 TBSP MINCED GARLIC

2 TBSP OLIVE OIL

1 TSP KOSHER SALT

4 TBSP LEMON JUICE

GRILLED VEGGIE SANDWICH

1 SMALL EGGPLANT, SLICED INTO STRIPS

1 SMALL ZUCCHINI, SLICED INTO STRIPS

1 SMALL YELLOW SQUASH, SLICED INTO STRIPS

2 LARGE PORTOBELLO MUSHROOMS

OLIVE OIL

SALT AND PEPPER TO TASTE

2 HEIRLOOM TOMATOES, SLICED

1 BUNCH BASIL, LEAVES PULLED

4 CIABATTA BUNS

1/2 CUP RICOTTA

JUICE OF 1 LEMON

1 GARLIC CLOVE MINCED

SALT AND PEPPER TO TASTE

PREPARATION

When ready to cook, set temperature to 180°F and preheat, lid closed for 15 minutes.

For the hummus: Drain and rinse the chickpeas and spread out on a sheet tray. Place tray in the grill grate and smoke for 15-20 minutes or to desired smoke level.

In the bowl of a food processor, combine smoked chickpeas, tahini, garlic, olive oil, salt and lemon juice and process until mixed well but not completely smooth. Transfer to a bowl and reserve.

Increase grill temp to high (400-500°F).

Toss eggplant, zucchini, squash, and portobellos with olive oil, lemon juice, salt and pepper. Place the veggies directly on the grill grate mushrooms gill side up. Cook veggies until grill marks develop and veggies are tender (10-15 minutes for sliced veggies, 20-25 min for mushrooms).

While the veggies are cooking combine the ricotta, lemon juice, garlic, salt and pepper in a small bowl.

Cut the ciabatta buns in half and open them up. Spread hummus on one side and ricotta on the other.

Stack the grilled veggies and top with tomatoes and basil. Enjoy!

ROASTED PICKLED BEETS

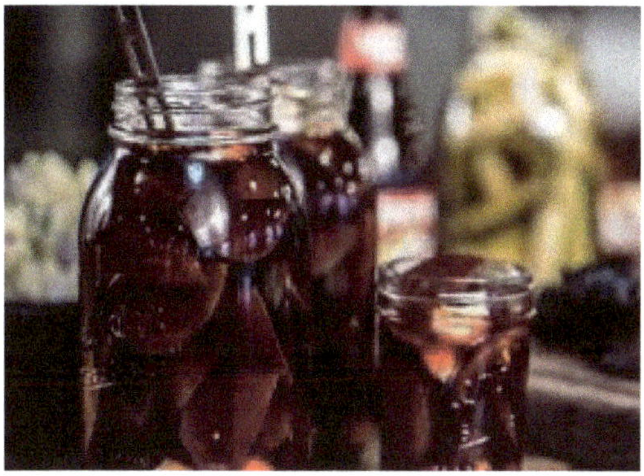

PREP TIME

15 MINS

COOK TIME

10 MINS

SERVES

8-12

HARDWOOD

MAPLE

INGREDIENTS

6 MEDIUM BEETS, PREFERABLY CANDY CANE BEETS, STEM ENDS TRIMMED

1 CUP HIGH-QUALITY RED WINE VINEGAR

1/2 CUP SUGAR OR HONEY

1 1/2 TSP. COARSE OR KOSHER SALT

1 CUP WATER

6-8 WHOLE CLOVES

5 WHOLE PEPPERCORNS

2 PIECES STAR ANISE

1 CINNAMON STICK, BROKEN IN HALF

PREPARATION

Make a foil pouch large enough to enclose the beets. Poke a few holes in the top to allow steam to escape.

When ready to cook, set the temperature to 350°F and preheat, lid closed for 15 minutes.

Roast the beets until they are tender, 50 to 60 minutes. Carefully remove the foil and allow the beets to cool until they can be comfortably handled.

Slip the skins off with your fingers. (You may wish to wear latex gloves to avoid staining your hands.)

Cut the beets into quarters or slices. (Candy cane beets are especially pretty when sliced.)

In the meantime, make the brine: Bring the vinegar, sugar, salt, and water to a boil in a small saucepan over high heat.

Put the cloves, peppercorns, star anise, and cinnamon in a clean lidded jar, such as a canning jar. Add the beets to the jar. Pour the hot brine over the beets. Put the lid on the jar. Cool the beets to room temperature, then refrigerate for 3 to 5 days before serving.

GRILLED ZUCCHINI SQUASH SPEARS

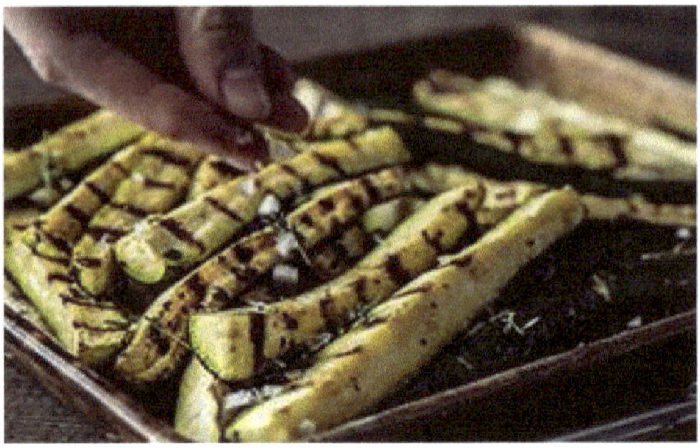

PREP TIME

5 MINS

COOK TIME

10 MINS

SERVES

4-6

HARDWOOD

OAK

INGREDIENTS

4 MEDIUM ZUCCHINI

2 TBSP OLIVE OIL

1 TBSP CHERRY VINEGAR

2 SPRINGS THYME, LEAVES PULLED

SALT AND PEPPER, TO TASTE

PREPARATION

Clean the zucchini and cut each end off. Cut each in half, then each half into thirds.

Combine remaining ingredients in a medium Ziploc bag and add the spears. Toss and mix well to coat the zucchini.

When ready to cook, set the temperature to 350°F and preheat, lid closed for 15 minutes.

Remove the spears form the bag and place directly on the grill grate cut side down.

Cook for 3-4 minutes per side, until grill marks appear and zucchini is tender.

Remove from grill and finish with more thyme leaves if desired.

Enjoy!

SMOKED PICKLED GREEN BEANS

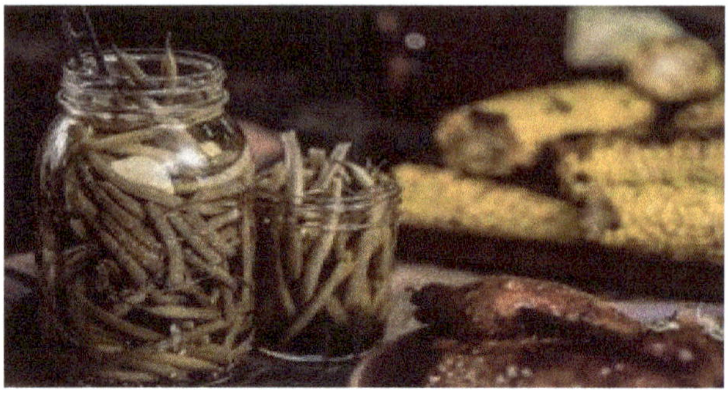

PREP TIME

15 MINS

COOK TIME

45 MINS

SERVES

4-6

HARDWOOD

OAK

INGREDIENTS

1 LB GREEN BEANS, BLANCHED

1/2 CUP SALT

1/2 CUP SUGAR

1 TBSP RED PEPPER FLAKE

2 CUPS WHITE WINE VINEGAR

2 CUPS ICE WATER

PREPARATION

*This requires overnight preparation.

When ready to cook, set temperature to 180°F and preheat, lid closed for 15 minutes.

Place the blanched green beans on a mesh grill mat and place mat directly on the grill grate. Smoke the green beans for 30-45 minutes until they've picked up the desired amount of smoke. Remove from grill and set aside until the brine is ready.

In a medium sized saucepan, bring all remaining ingredients, except ice water, to a boil over medium high heat on the stove. Simmer for 5-10 minutes then remove from heat and steep 20 minutes more. Pour brine over ice water to cool.

Once brine has cooled, pour over the green beans and weigh them down with a few plates to ensure they are completely submerged. Let sit 24 hours before use.

Enjoy!

SEAFOOD RECIPES FOR WOOD PELLET SMOKER GRILLS

GRILLED LOBSTER TAILS

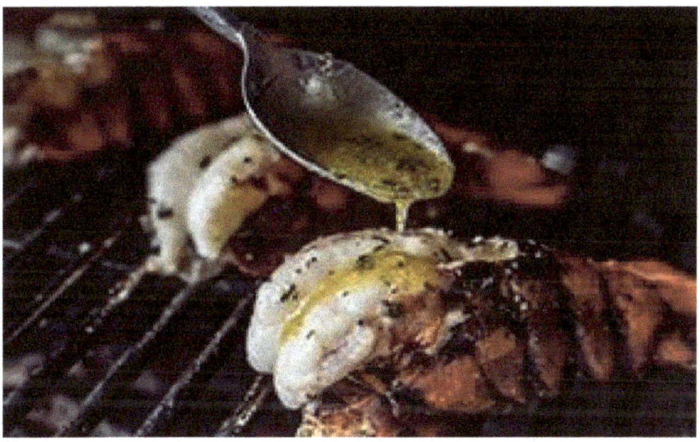

PREP TIME

10 MINS

COOK TIME

25 MINS

SERVES

2-4

HARDWOOD

OAK

INGREDIENTS

2 LOBSTER TAILS, 8-10 OZ EACH

8 TBSP BUTTER

2 TBSP LEMON JUICE

1 TSP PAPRIKA

1/4 TSP GARLIC SALT

1/4 TSP OLD BAY SEASONING

1/4 TSP FRESHLY GROUND BLACK PEPPER

2 TBSP FRESH PARSLEY, CHOPPED

PREPARATION

Prepare the lobster by cutting down the middle of the tough shell toward the tail with kitchen shears. Using your fingers, gently pry the meat from the shell, keeping it attached at the base of the tail. Lift the meat so it is resting on top of the split shell (again, keeping it attached at the base of the tail).

Make a slit down the middle of the meat to butterfly it open on top. Place the lobster tails on a rimmed baking sheet.

Melt the butter in a small saucepan over medium-low heat. Whisk in the lemon juice, paprika, garlic salt, Old Bay Seasoning, pepper, and parsley.

Pour about 1 tablespoon of the butter mixture over each lobster tail. Keep the remaining butter mixture warm.

When ready to cook, set temperature to High and preheat, lid closed for 15 minutes.

Remove the lobster tails from the baking sheet and arrange them directly on the grill grate. Cook for 25 to 30 minutes, or until the meat is white and opaque.

Transfer lobster tails to a platter and serve with the reserved butter mixture. Enjoy!

GARLIC SALMON

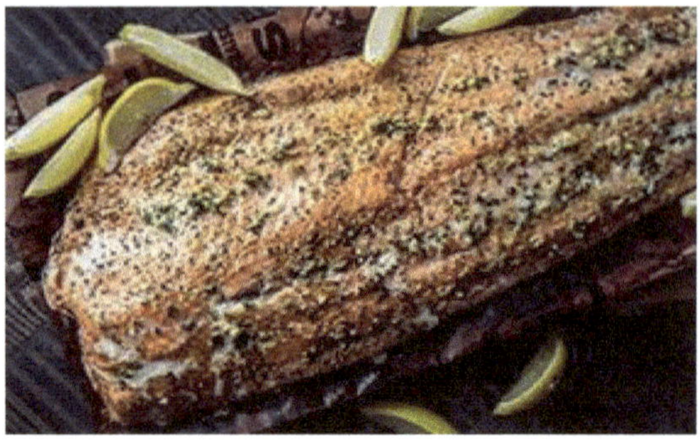

PREP TIME

5 MINS

COOK TIME

25 MINS

SERVES

4-6

HARDWOOD

ALDER

INGREDIENTS

1 2-3 LB SALMON FILET, SKIN ON

1/4 CUP OLIVE OIL

2 TBSP GARLIC, MINCED

1/2 TBSP PARSLEY, MINCED

TRAEGER FIN & FEATHER RUB

LEMON WEDGES, FOR SERVING

PREPARATION

Line a baking sheet with butcher paper or parchment. Place the salmon skin side down on the baking sheet and season the filet with the Traeger Fin & Feather Rub. In a small bowl combine olive oil, garlic, and parsley. Set aside.

When ready to cook, set temperature to High and preheat, lid closed for 15 minutes.

Brush the salmon with the garlic mixture and transfer the baking sheet to the grill. Cook until the internal temperature reaches 140°F (about 20-25 minutes), or until the fish flakes easily.

Remove from the grill and brush with any extra garlic mixture you may have and serve with lemon wedges.

Enjoy

GRILLED PANANG CURRY SALMON

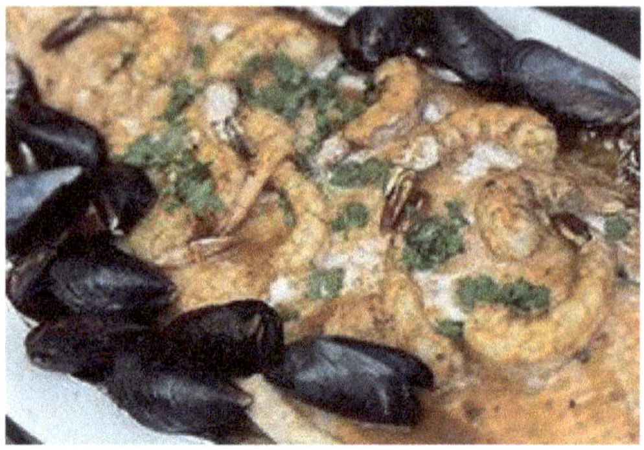

PREP TIME

35 MINS

COOK TIME

15 MINS

SERVES

2-4

HARDWOOD

ALDER

INGREDIENTS

PANANG CURRY SALMON

1 (12 OZ) JAR THAIFUSIONS PANANG CURRY

1 (4-7 LB) SALMON FILLET

2 SPRIGS THAI BASIL, ROUGHLY CHOPPED

1/2 RED BELL PEPPER SLICED THINLY, LENGTHWISE

1 LIME, SLICED INTO THIN CROSSCUT PIECES

MUSSELS WITH PRAWNS (OPTIONAL)

1/2 LB PRAWNS, SHELLED AND DEVEINED

1/2 LB MUSSELS DEBEARDED AND WASHED

HANDFUL THAI BASIL, CHOPPED

PREPARATION

Season both sides of the salmon with salt and pepper.

Brush a little canola oil on the salmon fillet and marinate with a 1/2 cup of Thaifusions Panang Curry in a shallow pan. Cover and marinate at room temperature for about 30 minutes.

When ready to cook, set temperature to High and preheat, lid closed for 15 minutes.

Brush some canola oil onto the grill so the salmon won't stick. Place salmon fillet directly on the grill grate and brush on about another 1/4 cup of

Thaifusions Panang Curry and top with sliced red bell pepper and lime slices.

Grill salmon until an internal temperature of 145°F, about 10-15 minutes.

For the Mussels and Prawns: Pour last 1/4 cup of Panang Curry into a sauce pan, add prawns, mussels, Thai basil and cover sauce pan and finish on the Traeger. When the mussels have opened, take off the grill and set aside.

Take salmon off the grill as gently as possible and top salmon with mussels and prawns if desired. Garnish with Thai basil. Enjoy!

SEARED LEMON GARLIC SCALLOPS

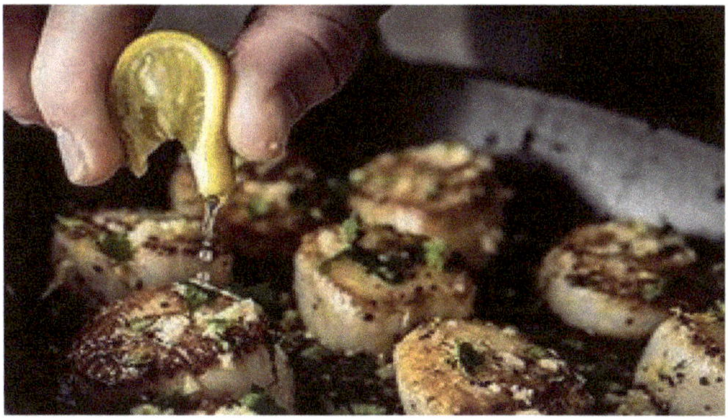

PREP TIME

5 MINS

COOK TIME

5 MINS

SERVES

4-6

HARDWOOD

ALDER

INGREDIENTS

SCALLOPS

1 DOZEN U-20 SCALLOPS

KOSHER SALT

1 TBSP BUTTER

1 TBSP OLIVE OIL

CHOPPED PARSLEY, TO GARNISH

LEMON ZEST, TO GARNISH

GARLIC BUTTER

4 TBSP BUTTER, MELTED

JUICE OF 1 LEMON

1 CLOVE GARLIC, MINCED

PREPARATION

When ready to cook, set the temperature to 400°F and preheat, lid closed for 15 minutes.

Remove the frill if it is still intact. Pat the scallops dry with a paper towel. Season liberally with salt and a bit of black pepper.

When the grill is hot, place the butter and olive oil on the skillet. When the butter has melted, place the scallops on the skillet. Close the lid and cook for about 2 minutes until seared and browned on one side.

While the scallops cook, combine the melted butter and garlic in a small bowl.

Flip the scallops, spoon a couple tablespoons of garlic butter over the top and cook for 1 minute longer.

Remove from the grill, add a little more garlic butter if desired and finish with parsley and lemon zest. Enjoy!

WHOLE GRILLED RED SNAPPER

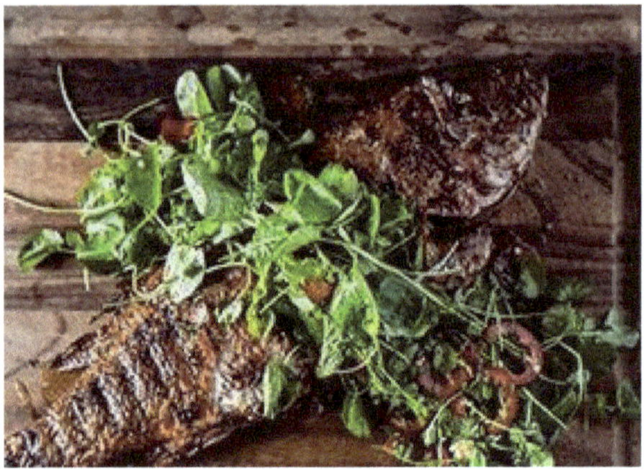

PREP TIME

10 MINS

COOK TIME

40 MINS

SERVES

1

HARDWOOD

MESQUITE

INGREDIENTS

RED SNAPPER

1 WHOLE RED SNAPPER, RINSE AND PAT DRY

2 TBSP OLIVE OIL

1/2 TBSP KOSHER SALT

1 TSP BLACK PEPPER

1/4 CUP BUTTER, MELTED

1/4 CUP HARISA

SALAD

1 BUNCH WATERCRESS, TRIMMED AND WASHED

2 CHERRY PEPPERS, THINLY SLICED

3 SCALLIONS, THINLY SLICED

2 TBSP CHOPPED CILANTRO

2 TBSP MINT LEAVES TORN

2 LIMES, JUICED

1 TSP BROWN SUGAR

1/4 TSP FISH SAUCE

1/4 CUP OLIVE OIL

SALT AND PEPPER, TO TASTE

PREPARATION

In a medium bowl combine melted butter and harissa.

When ready to cook, set the temperature to High and preheat, lid closed for 15 minutes.

Coat the exterior of the fish with olive oil and season with salt and pepper on both sides. Place fish directly on the grill grate, brush with the harissa-butter mixture and cook for 15-20 minutes.

While the fish cooks, prepare the salad. In a small bowl combine the lime juice, brown sugar, fish sauce, salt and pepper. While whisking, slowly stream in olive oil. In a medium bowl combine the watercress, peppers, scallions, cilantro and mint. Wait to dress the salad until ready to serve.

Flip the fish and brush the other side with harissa-butter mixture. Close the lid and continue to cook 10-15 minutes more until the internal temperature registers 145°F.

Carefully remove the fish from the grill and place on a serving platter. Drizzle the dressing over the greens, season to taste with salt and pepper and mix to coat.

Pile the salad over the top of the fish and drizzle the fish with remaining dressing if desired. Enjoy!

ROASTED HALIBUT IN PARCHMENT

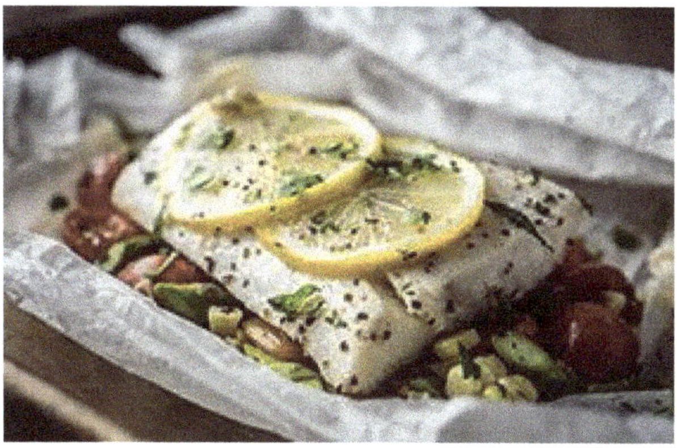

PREP TIME

15 MINS

COOK TIME

15 MINS

SERVES

4-6

HARDWOOD

ALDER

INGREDIENTS

4 EA (4 OZ) FISH FILLETS, SUCH AS SALMON, HALIBUT OR SNAPPER, PIN BONES REMOVED

EXTRA-VIRGIN OLIVE OIL

KOSHER SALT AND FRESHLY GROUND PEPPER

2 LEMONS, PREFERABLY MEYER, ENDS TRIMMED, CUT INTO 12 SLICES

KERNELS FROM 2 EARS OF CORN

16 ASPARAGUS SPEARS, BOTTOMS TRIMMED, SLICED INTO 1/2-INCH PIECES

2 TBSP FINELY CHOPPED ASSORTED HERBS, SUCH AS BASIL, CHIVES, OR PARSLEY

EQUIPMENT: 4 PIECES PARCHMENT PAPER

PREPARATION

When ready to cook, set the temperature to High and preheat, lid closed for 15 minutes.

Cut four pieces of parchment paper or Traeger butcher paper each 18" long.

Place a fish fillet on the center of a piece of parchment. Season with a pinch each of salt and pepper, then drizzle with olive oil. Place three lemon slices on the fillet, overlapping them slightly to cover the fish.

Sprinkle one-fourth each of the corn, asparagus, and tomatoes (if using) evenly around the fish, then drizzle with a little olive oil and season again with a small pinch each of salt and pepper.

Bring the long sides of the paper together, and fold the top edges down together to create a 1-inch seal, then continue to fold down tightly over the fish and vegetables.

Twist the open ends of the parchment in opposite directions to prevent steam from escaping.

Repeat the process with the remaining ingredients and parchment and place the packets on a baking sheet. If not cooking immediately, refrigerate for up to 4 hours.

Place the baking sheet on the Traeger and bake until the packets are lightly browned and have puffed up, about 15 minutes.

Transfer each packet to a plate and let stand for 5 minutes. Using sharp scissors, cut an X into the center of each packet and carefully pull back the parchment and sprinkle with the herbs.

Serve immediately. Enjoy!

GRILLED LOBSTER WITH LEMON GARLIC BUTTER RECIPE

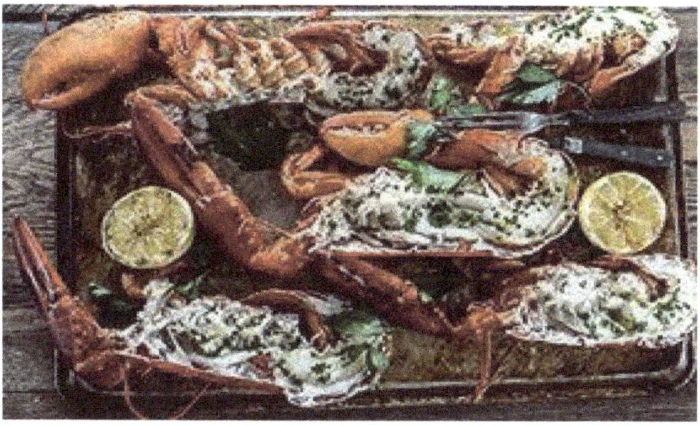

PREP TIME

10 MINS

COOK TIME

25 MINS

SERVES

4-6

HARDWOOD

HICKORY

INGREDIENTS

GRILLED LOBSTER

(4) 1 1/2 LB LIVE LOBSTERS

2 TBSP 2 T OLIVE OIL

2 LEMONS, SLICED

FLAT LEAF PARSLEY, TO SERVE

LEMON GARLIC BUTTER

3/4 CUP BUTTER, SOFTENED

2 TBSP FLAT LEAF PARSLEY, FINELY DICED

1 TBSP MINCED SHALLOT

2 CLOVES GARLIC, MINCED

1 TBSP LEMON JUICE

1 TBSP LEMON ZEST

1/2 TSP SEA SALT

1/2 TSP FRESH CRACKED BLACK PEPPER

PREPARATION

Bring a large stockpot of water to a rapid boil. Working in batches as necessary, submerge the lobster in the water head first, then cover with a lid. Cook for 5 minutes, then transfer to an ice-bath to cool and stop the cooking process.

In a small saucepan, melt the butter over medium low heat. When melted, add the remaining ingredients and whisk together until smooth. Set aside.

Using a very sharp knife, split the lobster into 2 halves. Clean out the tomalley from the body and discard. Brush the lobster halves all over with olive oil.

When ready to cook, set temperature to High and preheat, lid closed for 15 minutes.

When hot, place the lobsters on the grill, flesh side down, and cook for 4 minutes. Turn, and spoon about 2 tsp of compound butter onto each lobster halve. As the butter begins to melt, baste with a brush all over the flesh. Cook for 4-5 minutes until cooked through and coated in melted butter.

Serve immediately with sliced lemons and parsley. Enjoy!

BBQ OYSTERS

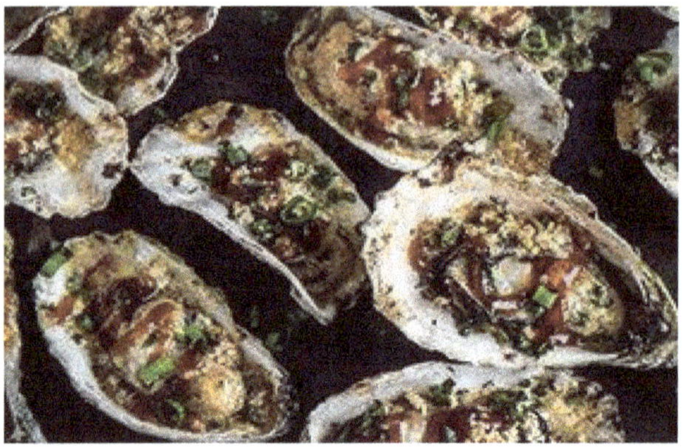

PREP TIME

10 MINS

COOK TIME

6 MINS

SERVES

4-6

HARDWOOD

APPLE

INGREDIENTS

BBQ OYSTERS

12 OYSTERS, SHUCKED

1 BUNCH GREEN ONIONS, CHOPPED

8 OZ SHREDDED PEPPER JACK CHEESE

1/4 CUP SEASONED BREAD CRUMBS

TRAEGER SWEET & HEAT BBQ SAUCE

COMPOUND BUTTER

1 LB BUTTER, UNSALTED

1 TBSP MEAT CHURCH THE GOSPEL OR HONEY HOG BBQ RUB

1/2 BUNCH GREEN ONIONS, MINCED

2 CLOVES GARLIC, MINCED

PREPARATION

When ready to cook, start the Traeger according to grill instructions. Set the temperature to 375 degrees F and preheat, lid closed, for 10 to 15 minutes.

For the compound butter: Allow the butter to soften. Combine butter, garlic, onion and BBQ Rub thoroughly.

Lay the butter on parchment paper or plastic wrap. Roll it up to form a log and tie each end with butcher's twine. Place in the freezer for an hour to solidify. You can use this butter on any grilled meats to enhance the flavor. You can also use a high-quality butter to replace the compound butter.

Shuck the oysters keeping all of the juice in the shell.

Sprinkle the oysters with bread crumbs and place directly on the Traeger. Cook them for 5 minutes. You will be looking for the edge of the oyster to start to curl slightly.

After 5 minutes place a spoonful of butter in the oysters. After the butter melts, add a pinch of pepper jack cheese.

Remove the oysters after 6 minutes on the grill total. Top oysters with a squirt of BBQ sauce and a few chopped onions. Allow to cool for 5 minutes, then enjoy!

SPICY SHRIMP SKEWERS

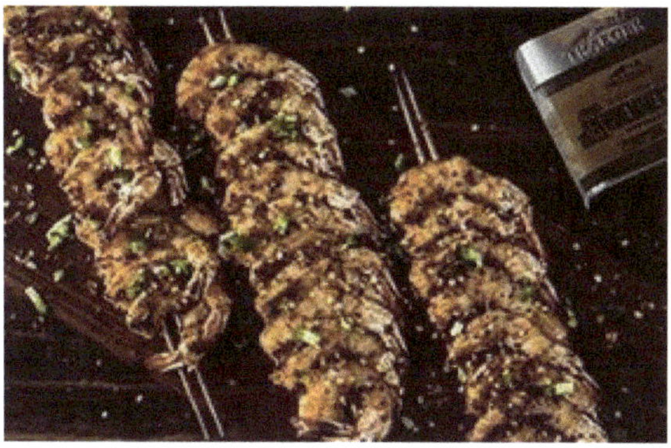

PREP TIME

10 MINS

COOK TIME

6 MINS

SERVES

4-6

HARDWOOD

APPLE

INGREDIENTS

2 LBS SHRIMP, PEELED, AND DEVEINED

6 OZ THAI CHILIES

6 CLOVES GARLIC

2 TBSP WINEMAKERS BLEND NAPA VALLEY RUB

1-1/2 TSP SUGAR

1-1/2 TBSP WHITE VINEGAR

3 TBSP OLIVE OIL

BAMBOO OR METAL SKEWERS

PREPARATION

Place all ingredients besides shrimp in a blender and blend until a course textured paste is reached.

Place shrimp in a bowl, add chili garlic mixture and place in fridge to marinate for at least 30 minutes.

Remove from fridge and thread shrimp onto bamboo or metal skewers.

When ready to cook, start the Traeger according to grill intructions. Set the temperature to 450 degrees F (set to 500 degrees F if using a WiFIRE enables grill) and preheat, lid closed, for 10 to 15 minutes.

Place shrimp on grill and cook for 2 to 3 minutes per side or until shrimp are pink and firm to touch. Enjoy!

BAJA-STYLE FISH TACOS

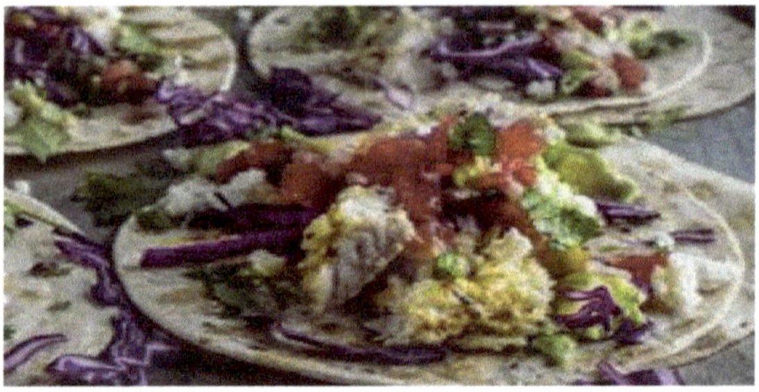

PREP TIME

10 MINS

COOK TIME

20 MINS

SERVES

4-6

HARDWOOD

APPLE

INGREDIENTS

1 LB. WHITE FISH SUCH AS COD, MONKFISH, OR HALIBUT (SKINLESS)

2 LIMES

2 TSP. DIJON-STYLE MUSTARD

1/2 TSP. SALT

1/2 TSP. BLACK PEPPER, FRESHLY GROUND

1/2 CUP VEGETABLE OIL, OR OLIVE OIL

2 CLOVES GARLIC, MINCED

AS NEEDED TRAEGER CAJUN RUB

8 CORN TORTILLAS

FOR SERVING SHREDDED CABBAGE, DICED RED ONIONS, CILANTRO LEAVES, PICKLED JALAPENO SLICES, DICED AVACADO, PICO DE GALLO OR SALSA, SOUR CREAM

PREPARATION

Juice one lime. Cut the other lime in wedges; set aside until serving time.

Make the marinade: In a small mixing bowl, combine the lime juice, mustard, and salt and pepper. Slowly whisk in the oil, then stir in the garlic.

Place the fish in a resealable plastic bag, pour the marinade over it, and refrigerate for no more than 1 hour.

When ready to cook, start the Traeger grill on Smoke with the lid open until the fire is established (4 to 5 minutes). Set the temperature to 400F (High on a 3-position controller) and preheat, lid closed, for 10 to 15 minutes.

Remove the fish from the marinade and pat off any excess marinade with paper towels. Season generously on both sides with Traeger Cajun Rub.

Arrange the fish on the grill grate and grill until the fish is opaque and flakes easily when pressed with a fork. (There is no need to turn it.) Remove to a cutting board and cut into bite-size chunks. Meanwhile, warm the tortillas on the Traeger until pliant and hot.

Arrange the fish, tortillas, and suggested accompaniments on a large platter. Garnish with the reserved lime wedges. Serve immediately enjoy.

I HOPE YOU FIND THE 100 RECIPES WOOD PELLET SMOKER GRILLS HELPFUL!!!

CPSIA information can be obtained
at www.ICGtesting.com
Printed in the USA
LVHW071147231120
672397LV00032B/1594

9 781801 128148